PRESIDENTIAL HEALTH MATTERS

PRESIDENTIAL HEALTH MATTERS

THE MEDICAL HISTORY OF THE UNITED STATES AS SEEN THROUGH THE LIVES OF FORTY-SIX PRESIDENTS

EDWARD LEWIS GOLDBERG, MD

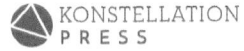

Copyright © 2023 by Edward Lewis Goldberg, MD

All rights reserved.

Konstellation Press, San Diego

www.konstellationpress.com

No part of this book may be reproduced in any form or by any electronic or mechanical means, including information storage and retrieval systems, without written permission from the author, except for the use of brief quotations in a book review.

Editor: Martin Roy Hill

Cover Design: Scarlet Willette

Author photo: Rowena Lomboy

Cover image: Professors Welch, Halsted, Osler and Kelly, aka The Four Doctors, by John Singer Sargent, 1906; Johns Hopkins University, (Baltimore)

ISBN: 979-8-9868432-0-9

To the memory of the thousands of health care workers, who gave up their lives during Covid 19

CONTENTS

Prologue	1
Introduction	3
1. The Impact of Viral Disease upon American History	11
2. Frontier Medicine Helps Build a Nation	38
3. The Long Gun—Legend Becomes Fact	48
4. The Impact of Viral Disease upon American History—From the Atlantic to the Pacific	54
5. Great Men, Great Women, Great Ideas	71
6. The Transfer of Presidential Power	88
7. Parade of Presidents	93
8. The Killing of James Garfield, or "Ignorance is Bliss"	116
9. Tale of Two Paintings	129
10. Less than best medical care	137
11. Presidential Cover-ups; Privacy and Assorted Sins and Misdemeanors	150
12. Benefits of Hospitalization	160
13. Pandemics: Wilson and Trump, Lessons not Learned	174
14. Disaster in Paris 1919, Stalemate in the US Senate	190
15. Franklin Delano Roosevelt	205
16. "How Ike Beat Heart Disease and Held onto the Presidency"	225
17. The Agony of Jack Kennedy, JFK (1917-1963)	241
18. The Shooting of Ronald Reagan, and the Triumph of US Medicine	276
Epilogue	287
Endnotes	293
Glossary	335
List of images and attributions	343
Bibliography	347
Acknowledgments	349
About the Author	355

PROLOGUE

My muse for this interest in medical history was the late Dr. Pasquale (Pat) Genovese.

I was fortunate to be a medical resident who reveled in his tales of the great doctors of the past. Pat told the following story: "While serving as a medical officer with the British 8th Army during WWII, the cardiologist, Dr. Paul Wood returned at night to his tent in the North African desert and wrote his classic cardiology textbook. An epiphany came to Wood one night, the description of the EKG changes of acute *pericarditis*, a benign disease of the heart. Accordingly, he recorded these changes in his manuscript."

A few years later, while caring for a patient with chest pains, I watched similar changes evolve on EKG tracings over several days. "My patient does not have a heart attack, it's only pericarditis." This was an experience a young doctor does not forget. I became hooked on the history of medicine, especially when there were such important lessons to be learned.

At age 82, Dr. John Bumgarner wrote *The Health of the Presidents,* which was a mother lode of information for me. This volume inspired me at the relatively young age of 79 to try my hand at writing a medical history. Dr. Bumgarner's book was my final authority on several occasions. But I have written a different book than Dr. Bumgarner. I have recycled or re-used similar or familiar threads to weave a new tapestry, focused upon medical and political history and the consequences of disease upon political history. This book is told in my voice and in my words.

INTRODUCTION

Along the highway of history looms the dangerous intersection of medical science and presidential politics. Many chose to ignore the flashing yellow warning lights. Consequently, the landscape has been littered with the wreckage of their collisions. The Battle of the Covid Pandemic is the latest manifestation of the collision between science and politics. The Prize of the Battle: Whose truth will prevail?

In this book, events of medical progress will be matched with the political events that happened at the same time. The effect of medical events upon US political history has been profound. Conversely, the health of some of the US presidents has also had an impact upon historical events. To paraphrase Tolstoy, some presidents were in the saddle directing the flow of history while other presidents would be passengers swept along by the flow of history.

Scientific progress had a great impact upon the medical care and health of the presidents. Their health improved with the advent of modern medicine and surgery. Presidents Thomas Jefferson and Theodore Roosevelt (TR) channeled their knowledge of medicine and science to bend the flow of history toward their political goals. They were able to utilize their knowledge of medical events for their political advantage. (Louisiana Purchase, Panama Canal).

Franklin Delano Roosevelt (FDR) and Lyndon Johnson also made major contributions to medical care, the March of Dimes and Medicare.[1] Unfortunately Presidents Woodrow Wilson and Donald Trump also had major impact upon medical care but in a negative way. Neither one was fully engaged with leading the fight against the Influenza epidemic of 1918 nor the Covid 19 epidemic of 2020.[2] Those failures led to disaster for the world.

Wilson and FDR also became ill at critical times, at Paris in 1919 and at Yalta in 1945. As a result, the Western world suffered diplomatic disasters.

The growth of science can be seen as a continuum, with each generation expanding upon the knowledge of their predecessors. This march of science was accelerated by occasional bursts of genius, such as Newton, Darwin, and Einstein. As explained by Isaac Newton, "If I have seen further than others, it is by standing upon the shoulders of giants."[3] Overall, the march of science in the US progressed in step with the march of the non-Native American people (the Americans) across the continent. The growth of the American empire from coast to coast and around the globe was greatly affected by medical events.

The structure of the book will be similar to a tapestry, woven together from many threads, as warp and weft. The warp will be the longitudinal threads that will flow from top to bottom from past to present. Each warp thread carries a unique list of historical events: the sequential list of the presidents, and the history of medical progress from the Greek philosophers to genomes.

The weft will be the horizontal threads carrying the themes

included in the book: i.e. incompetent medical care, presidential disability, the rise of hospitals, medical cover-ups, and the maintenance of a peaceful political transition between successive presidents.

As a horizontal thread (weft) moves across the loom from left to right, it intersects with a longitudinal thread. Each intersection becomes the locus for one of the stories of the book, i.e., the assassination of President James Garfield. At this location, the threads of the germ theory had intersected with the threads of post-Civil War politics.

The shuttle is controlled by the scribe, who weaves the threads into a story. It does not show chaos, but rather an intricate web of connectedness between many different events and stories which represent the intersections of the threads. Seemingly disparate events will be shown to be related.

Does the scribe direct the stream of events according to a preconceived outlook? After all, the scribe chooses what threads to pick up, and which ones to discard. Or does the scribe follow the flow of events, allowing the readers to make their own determination as to what happened?

This book also serves as a travelogue to help us find our way through time, focused upon the years 1721 to 2021: from the struggle to control smallpox in Boston to the disastrous Covid 19 pandemic.[4] Please consider as introductory any comments about events prior to 1775.

The **TIMELINE** graph represents a more linear presentation of the medical and political events that make up this tapestry.

The presidents are listed in chronological order along the left-hand vertical axis. Each president is followed by their years in office. The right-hand vertical column represents medical events contemporaneous with that president's time in office.

TIMELINE:

President	Term	Event	Year
George Washington	1789-1797	William Jenner begins inoculation with cowpox	1796
John Adams	1797-1801	Death of Washington	1799
Thomas Jefferson	1801-1809	Yellow Fever in Haiti	1801
James Madison	1809-1817	Ephraim McDowell does first abdominal surgery	1809
James Monroe	1817-1825	McDowell operates upon James K Polk	1816
John Quincy Adams	1825-1829	Louis Pierre begins statistical analysis of medicine	1828
Andrew Jackson	1829-1837	Oliver Wendell Holmes studies with Louis Pierre	1833
Martin van Buren	1837-1841	"Experiments and Observations on…Gastric Juice"	1838
William H. Harrison	1841-1841	Died on the 30th day of his presidency	1841
John Tyler	1841-1845	Crawford Long begins to use ether anesthesia	1842
James Polk	1845-1849	Semmelweis lowers death rate from puerperal sepsis	1848
Zachary Taylor	1849-1850	Last president treated with Heroic Therapy	1850
Millard Fillmore	1850-1853	Claude Bernard begins his PhD at the Sorbonne	1850
Franklin Pierce	1853-1857	John Snow and the Broad St water pump handle	1854
James Buchanan	1857-1861	Charles Darwin publishes "Origin of the Species"	1859
Abraham Lincoln	1861-1865	US Sanitary Commission created	1861
Andrew Johnson	1865-1869	First gall-bladder surgery in US	1867
US Grant	1869-1877	Joseph Lister tours the US	1876
Rutherford B. Hayes	1877-1881	Louis Pasteur isolates the microbe Pasteurella	1878
James Garfield	1881-1881	Pasteur developed vaccine for anthrax	1881
Chester Arthur	1881-1885	Koch develops TB bacillus	1882
Grover Cleveland	1885-1889	Yellow fever drives French out of Panama	1889
Benjamin Harrison	1889-1893	Anti-toxin used to treat and cure diphtheria	1892
Grover Cleveland	1893-1897	Wilhelm Roentgen discovers the Xray	1895
William McKinley	1897-1901	Walter Reed shows mosquito bite causes YF	1901
Theodore Roosevelt	1901-1909	Willem Einthoven invents the EKG	1903
William H. Taft	1909-1913	Flexner report issued	1910
Woodrow Wilson	1913-1921	The Influenza Pandemic begins	1918
Warren Harding	1921-1923	Banting and Best discover insulin.	1921
Calvin Coolidge	1923-1929	Alexander Fleming discovers penicillin	1928
Herbert Hoover	1929-1933	First cardiac catheterization	1929
Franklin Roosevelt	1939-1945	Dr. D. Harkins removes bullets from the hearts of 134 US army soldiers, and they all survived	1944
Harry Truman	1945-1953	Sidney Farber begins to use cancer chemotherapy	1946
Dwight Eisenhower	1953-1961	Reserpine, first anti Hypertension drug in use	1954
John Kennedy	1961-1963	First coronary care units are built	1962
Lyndon Johnson	1963-1969	Medicare bill becomes law	1965
Richard Nixon	1969-1974	Clean Water Act becomes law	1972
Gerald Ford	1974-1977	Swine Flu outbreak	1976
Jimmy Carter	1977-1981	Last known case smallpox (outside labs)	1977
Ronald Reagan	1981-1989	AIDS epidemic begins	?1981
George H.W. Bush	1889-1993	Genome project begins	1990
Bill Clinton	1993-2001	Clinton refuses to destroy smallpox stores.	1999
George W. Bush	2001-2009	US Capitol attacked with anthrax spores	2001
Barack Obama	2009-2017	Epidemic Zika virus disease Puerto Rico	2016
Donald Trump	2017-2021	Covid RNA vaccine developed	2020

Timeline of Presidents

At times the vertical lines were not synchronous and tension occurred. This is best exemplified by the entrenched opposition to the germ theory of infectious disease that lasted until the 1880s, despite the published works of Jenner, Semmelweis, Lister, Pasteur and Koch. The cultural descendants of these germ theory opponents can be found in today's anti-maskers, and the anti-vaccine movement that has continued to plague the nation since 1721.

Prior to 1912, the overall impact of medical intervention upon patients was negative. Examples were bloodletting and toxic medical therapy employing heavy metals. The tipping point occurred around 1912, and medical intervention thereafter was likely to have a positive outcome.[5] This came about by the control of infectious diseases by early vaccines, widespread application of filtered municipal drinking water, control of mosquitoes, and the rise of public health. Childbirth became safer, surgical infections were less frequent and effective anesthesia allowed surgery to be tolerable. Hospitals became uncrowded, clean, and well ventilated.

The highlight was the Flexner report of 1910 that had reformed medical education. US doctors were now beginning to be well trained.[6] The health of the public, including the presidents, benefited from all of these changes.

Medical care for American Presidents.

About one third of all the presidents have been seriously ill during their presidency, and the response to their illnesses was uneven and unsatisfactory. Some presidents, like Garfield received incompetent medical care, while others like Ronald Reagan, received excellent care. The unresolved issue is there is still no way to assure that the president is receiving excellent medical care.

Since 1789 the issue of presidential privacy remains unresolved. We assume that the public has a right to know about the president's health, since an informed public is required in a democracy. However, the practice of the presidents since the time of Chester Arthur has been to cover-up their ailments. For Grover Cleveland, the cover-up was truly spectacular, and involved secret surgery on a yacht sailing up the East River in New York City.

In 2023, John F. Kennedy's medical history continues to be hidden from the public fifty-nine years after his death in 1963. This is worrisome because JFK's cover-ups may also have endangered the world during the Cuban Missile Crisis.

Other presidents besides Kennedy have been involved in attempts to cover up ailments. and disabilities. Most of these coverups were created to maintain political power (Cleveland, FDR) and had little to do with privacy issues. The public was not well-served. However, since Eisenhower's time most presidents except Kennedy and Trump chose to inform the public of their health and surrendered a lot of privacy in doing so.

Since the first days of the Republic, medicine and presidential politics have been inextricably linked. Donald Trump was ill with Covid-19 and received non-standard care from his physician, who did not disclose the critical details of Trump's illness. That apparently supported Trump's attempts to downplay the significance of the pandemic.

The mixing of politics and presidential mental health has always been a difficult task for physicians, politicians, and historians. Several presidents have had mental health issues, including three who had significant clinical depression: Franklin Pierce, Abraham Lincoln, and Calvin Coolidge, and of the three only Lincoln was fully functional.

The apparent egomania and mendacity of Donald Trump are worrisome but may not necessarily be the signs of a mental illness. Just prior to his resignation in 1974, Richard Nixon was seen to be wandering through the White House speaking to the portraits that hung on the walls. This was probably the one-time act of a man facing ruin. It is not necessary to consider an underlying mental disease.[7]

There is a need to separate illness from the concept of disability. FDR was not disabled from polio, but he was disabled from heart failure.

But it will be the overlap of these issues, i.e, when a disabled president hides his illness from the public that great harm is done. That occurred in 1919 when for seventeen months the US had no functioning president. The result was a disaster for the US and the world.

What can be learned from the issues of the past? Avoid the repetition of errors but support those decisions that went well. Hopefully, the lessons of history will help us to navigate the future. Let's see how that has played out over the years.

1
THE IMPACT OF VIRAL DISEASE UPON AMERICAN HISTORY

Smallpox, the Speckled Monster: "*A virus is a bunch of bad news surrounded by a protein,*" attributed to Sir Peter Medawar, Nobel laureate of 1960

1A. BRIEF WORLD history of smallpox:

Smallpox was a critical factor in the European settlement of the Americas. It also played a major role in the events of the American Revolution. Accordingly, it is appropriate to discuss smallpox in detail. The response of the 18th century public to the smallpox vaccine foreshadowed American reactions to all future vaccines. This has been an ongoing issue in American history. It has separated those who believe in science from those who do not, and has had huge consequences.

Viral epidemics had a great impact upon the European settlement of the Americas and the expansion of the American empire. Both George Washington and Thomas Jefferson played major roles in that story.

Smallpox is caused by a virus, but that term was not in use

until the end of the nineteenth century. Nor had anyone ever seen a virus until the introduction of the electron microscope in 1931. Despite those drawbacks, 18th and 19th century scientists were able to control smallpox, Yellow Fever, and rabies; all three are viral illness. This demonstrated the power of abstract thinking, intuitive thought, and the genius of Edward Jenner, Carlos Finlay, William Gorgas, and Louis Pasteur.

Smallpox was well documented in Egyptian hieroglyphics for over 3,000 years. The pox were seen on the face of the mummy of Rameses V, who died in 1145 BCE. His tomb was uncovered in 1898.

However, smallpox did not appear in Europe until the 6th century C.E. and did not appear in the New World until the 16th century with the arrival of the Europeans. The Spaniards were probably the first, but not the last, to bring small pox to the New World. This occurred by way of infected soldiers, sailors, missionaries, traders, explorers, and settlers who crossed the ocean and infected the natives they encountered upon landing in the Americas.[1]

The Native Americans reciprocated for the gift of smallpox with a similar gift for the Europeans. When the Spaniards returned to Europe in 1493, they brought syphilis back with them.[2] There is no definitive evidence that syphilis existed in Europe before then.[3]

However, it was smallpox that played the critical role in the European settlement of the New World. Its effect upon the Native Americans was devastating, since they never had any prior exposure and had never acquired any immunity to smallpox.

When Columbus landed on the island of Hispaniola in 1492 there were estimated to be hundreds of thousands of Native Americans (Tainos) on the island.

In 1507 the Spaniards did the first census on Hispaniola and recorded about 60,000 living Tainos. That population loss was due to forced labor and starvation, ongoing warfare, and intermarriage with Spaniards. Similar events would occur throughout the Americas for the next several hundred years.

In 1518 smallpox was first recorded on Hispaniola and it was observed that most of the remaining Tainos began to succumb to this disease. For the next several hundred years smallpox became the leading cause of death among the indigenous Americans.

By 1531 there were only 600 Tainos still alive on Hispaniola, only 1 percent of the 1507 census.

This is evidence for the destruction of the Tainos by smallpox.[4] There was a 99 per cent death rate in only 24 years. That experience can be extrapolated to the rest of North and South America, since there was similar evidence for other tribes at other times and places with similar collapse of the population following introduction to smallpox.

How many indigenous people lived in the pre-Colombian New World (Americas) is a challenging question. One estimate for the year 1500 has 100 million natives living in the New World, with about one third of them north of the Rio Grande.

By 1700, 200 years later, there were only about five million Native Americans left, with only about one million living north of the Rio Grande. Small pox was the major culprit for this decline. There may have been other causes for this decline, including measles, but these are not as well documented.[5]

By 1775, as the United States began to expand beyond the Appalachian Mountains, the pioneers came across a relatively empty, sparsely populated North American continent. The people who used to live there were gone, wiped out by smallpox. This was similar to all the empty apartment houses in Berlin in 1941, that had been owned by German Jews, deported or murdered by the Nazis.

From President Jackson until President Grant, the US had a very poor record of providing protection for Native Americans. Thankfully, President Grant ended the policy of killing Native Americans, and began placing them on relatively safer reservations.[6] The slaughter of thousands of innocents finally ended, but the population was decimated. The 1890 US census estimated that only 250,000 Native Americans were left in the US. Following Grant's leadership the wholesale murder had stopped, the Native Americans were in a safer place, and extinction was reversed. The 2020 US Census now lists 9.7 million American Indians and Alaska Natives, almost three percent of the total US population. For many years, the experts had ranked Grant as the worst of all presidents. The prevention of genocide apparently didn't fit into their ranking algorithm.

TRANSMISSION OF SMALLPOX is usually human to human, by coughing or sneezing infected respiratory droplets onto the victim. Smallpox can also be transmitted from contact with dried scabs and dried secretions on paper and cloth, and especially infected blankets. There is no animal nor insect *vector* involved in smallpox. Nor can the disease be spread by contaminated food or water.

During the 17th and 18th centuries, smallpox was relatively common in Europe and North America, and was endemic with sporadic cases. Epidemics occurred at unpredictable intervals and were usually associated with a mortality above thirty percent. Death from toxemia could occur at any time during the course of the disease. There was a lower death rate of about twenty percent in non-epidemic years. Surviving patients had complete resolution of all their symptoms and recovered fully by about day thirty. Survivors were *immune* for life against a recurrence of smallpox.

Knowledge of smallpox transmission led to three horrible uses of smallpox virus.

1. The awareness of the respiratory transmission of smallpox led the British army in North America to

employ sick prisoners, deserters, and slaves as biological weapons. These sick humans were sent into enemy lines in order to spread disease.
2. The British traded infected blankets with Native Americans for the purpose of killing them. They knew the blankets of smallpox victims were contagious, and those that came in contact with them were at risk of contracting smallpox. This was genocide.
3. After World War II, the US and the USSR built smallpox bombs, explosive weapons dropped from airplanes to disperse living smallpox virus in order to infect the people below. There is no evidence that these bombs have been destroyed.[8]

The letters of Lord Jeffrey Amherst, July 1763, advocated the policy of sending smallpox infected blankets to Native Americans and are evidence that the ensuing death were not accidental.[7] Imagine naming a college or your hometown after a man who was an advocate of genocide. In Canada and New Zealand, geographical places are now being restored to the original indigenous names. Maybe Massachusetts will follow suit.

We can understand what makes smallpox such a major killer by looking at the three phases of smallpox. And that will first require some definitions. The Merriam-Webster Dictionary defines:

Infectious as a property of microorganisms that are capable of invading and multiplying in body tissues. The root word is invade. Something can be infectious without being contagious, e.g. bacterial food poisoning.

Contagious as capable of being transmitted from person to person, communicable is a synonym. The root word is contact.

Phase 1. Small pox has a long incubation period of 10 to 12 days. There are no symptoms during this phase. That allows an infected but not yet contagious person to travel far and wide.

The disease could spread as far as an infected person could travel in 12 days.

Phase 2. The incubation period is followed by about one to two days of minimal symptoms before the pox erupt and present themselves as a warning to others. This second phase is *contagious* and dangerous to others. However, because of absence of any pox, a phase 2 infected person might not be recognized and, therefore, might not be quarantined.

Phase 3. During the final 18 to 20 days, patients have fever, pox and cough, and remain *contagious* until the last pox is gone. These patients are readily seen as being infected. They are very sick, bed-ridden, and unable to care for themselves.

There are special problems that occur in caring for them.[9] Twenty days is a long time for an infected person to be spewing their contagious particles into the air around caregivers and others. The caregivers were at great risk of infection, unless they were smallpox survivors. The virus also remained viable on patient's bedding, bandages and clothes, and their disposal was problematic.

The last remaining pox might be difficult to see, hidden in an armpit, behind the knee, lower back etc. The patient might erroneously think they were free of the pox, when they were not. So, with a false sense of security, a still contagious person might go out into society and continue to infect others.

The thirty-day length for each case of smallpox explains how smallpox could cross the Atlantic in the 16th century. The length of the trans-Atlantic journey was quite variable, an average of eighty days, with a range of twenty to ninety days. The virus could endure on board ship no matter the duration of the time at sea by spreading from person to person on board, from the time of departure to the time of arrival. An infected traveler in phase 2 or phase 3 could land on shore in North America and begin the process of infecting any Native Americans they met.[10]

Since the natives were a virgin group without any smallpox

immunity, the disease exploded through the native population. That is why the population of natives collapsed so dramatically.

Introduction to smallpox kept re-occurring over 300 years, everywhere in the New World that the Europeans landed and traveled, from Arctic Canada to Patagonia. This explains the collapse of the population everywhere in the New World, especially at First Contact.[12]

Over 50,000 slave ships crossed the Atlantic to the New World in the 16th, 17th, and 18th centuries.[11] There were also thousands of ship crossings for European traders and settlers. Each landing was another opportunity to spread smallpox to Native Americans.

When Queen Anne of England died in 1714, the Stuart Dynasty came to an end. Despite seventeen pregnancies, she had no surviving children. Four of her children, including her last living child and heir to the throne, died of smallpox and Anne was herself a smallpox survivor. The British nobility then turned to Germany and the House of Hanover for the next Protestant royal family of Great Britain. So, the royal family and the aristocracy had great interest in the control of smallpox in order to provide stability for the royal succession.[13]

Lady Mary Montagu was a friend of Queen Anne. She was a writer, and a very well-connected aristocrat who was also friends with the poet Alexander Pope and the politician Horace Walpole. In December 1715, she contracted smallpox that left her with deeply pitted skin, ruining her good looks. Her personal involvement deepened when, eighteen months later, smallpox infected and killed her twenty-year-old brother.

In 1717, her husband was named British ambassador to the Ottoman Empire and Lady Montagu and their children accompanied him to Constantinople. While there, Lady Montagu witnessed variolation. This involved taking infected material from a smallpox-infected person and injecting it under the skin of the arm of a healthy person. This transfer was done with a needle or a thorn.

If variolation was successful, the recipients were protected from getting the smallpox disease. Recipients almost always became ill with fever and pox, usually very mild. They were also contagious for a while. This point became a crucial factor for the American Revolution and the Continental Army. Newly inoculated soldiers were too sick to fight and were also contagious for a period of time.

While still in Constantinople, Lady Montagu had her son Edward undergo successful variolation. Upon her return to England, Lady Montagu introduced the details of variolation, and had her four-year-old daughter variolated in the presence of the physicians of the Royal court.

Unfortunately, about two percent of variolation recipients contracted a fatal case of smallpox. But Dr. Hans Sloan, president of the Royal Society and the Royal College of Physicians, and another powerful advocate for variolation, claimed that by employing shallow *intra-dermal* injections, the death rate was reduced to 0.3 percent.

A death rate from 0.3 to 2 percent for variolation was somewhat acceptable during an epidemic, but less so during non-epidemic years. So, the application of variolation was not uniform in time or place throughout England. However, Lady Montagu maintained her interest in smallpox and remained an influential advocate for variolation. As a result of her efforts, variolation was adopted by the Royal Family to protect the succession of the Hanovers, and by the nobility, the rich and powerful, the educated and the elite and, for the purposes of our story, by the British Army.[14]

New England had periodic smallpox epidemics in the 1600s and again in 1702. Between epidemics, smallpox persisted, but at lower rates. In 1721, a smallpox epidemic was once again raging in Boston. The Puritan minister Cotton Mather watched three of his own children come down with the disease. Mather then learned of the ancient practice of smallpox inoculation from his slave, Onesimus, a native of what is now southern Libya. Mather asked, "Have you ever had smallpox?"

"Yes and no" replied the slave. In those three words were the essence of variolation. Onesimus had been inoculated as a child in Africa and that inoculation had been followed by a mild case of smallpox. Onesimus informed Mather about this inoculation, a procedure practiced throughout Africa for centuries, and identical to the variolation method of Mary Montagu.

Mather urged local doctors to begin performing variolation against the disease. Against hostile public opinion, Dr. Zabdiel Boylston agreed to try the technique, beginning with his only son. This daring experiment rested directly on the testimony of a slave.

During the epidemic, Mather and Boylston kept a record of their findings.

- In 1721 the population of Boston was about 11,000.
- The number of small pox cases in Boston was 5,889.
- The incidence of smallpox during Boston epidemic was 5,889/11000 or 54%.
- The number of smallpox deaths in the city in 1721 was 844.
- The overall city-wide death rate from smallpox was 844/11000 or 8%.
- The death rate for people who had smallpox was 844/5889 or 14%.

How do those rates of death compare with the brave Bostonians who received variolation?

There were 287 people who received variolation, and six of them died. So, the death rate of people receiving variolation was 6/287 or 2 percent.

This is the first reported use of numbers to evaluate a clinical trial anywhere in the world. It showed the apparent protection of variolation during a smallpox epidemic. Those residents who received variolation had the best chance for survival during the smallpox epidemic of 1721.[15]

For his efforts during the 1721 epidemic, Mather has been called "the first significant figure in American medicine." He was the first colonial American to become a member of the Royal Society of London, and he wrote over 400 publications in his lifetime. Unfortunately for his place in history, he wrote one book too many, *The Wonders of the Invisible World*, a volume that supported the Salem Witch Trials.[16]

An angry mob in Boston responded to the 1721 variolation by firebombing Dr. Boylston's home. Contrast that Boston experience with the greater acceptance to variolation in England. Resistance to variolation in North America continued to be widespread, that was not surprising, considering the population's growing disdain for royal decrees and acts of Parliament.

This difference had dramatic consequences in the Revolutionary War, and this anti-vaccine sentiment continued in the US, re-emerging with deep-throated fury as the anti-masking, anti-vaccine campaign of 2020-2022

Variolation improved with the Sutton method, discovered in the 1760s. This method used the pus from other inoculated patients and not from primary patients. There was less morbidity, and the procedure was probably just as effective. Accordingly, there was a small renewal in variolation. Patients still needed to be quarantined after Sutton's variolation, because they were contagious until they were clear of skin lesions.

In 1776 the smallpox epidemic in North America involved the city of Boston. Abigail Adams and her children had never been inoculated. She travelled from Braintree to Boston to have the family inoculated by Dr. Thomas Bullfinch. Abigail had kept herself informed and was pro active.

Shortly after being variolated, Abigail Adams allegedly went walking in public. Her critics cried that "she was endangering the poor by exposing them to her pustules." This may have been an early example of misinformation, deliberate or otherwise. On July 18, 1776 a few days after being inoculated she went to the Old State House in Boston to hear the first public reading of the Declaration of Independence. She had no pox or pustules on her skin, so the accusation that she went about the public spreading her pustules is false. She was probably infectious but not contagious.

The Massachusetts Historical Society states that Mrs. Adams and her children remained in isolation for two months until all her children's inoculations were complete, the visit to the Old State House being the only exception. She was fulfilling her patriotic duty. No matter the reasons, concerns about science and medicine were splitting along along class lines. This was not the last time there appeared to be special rules for the elite.

The 1721 epidemic in Boston demonstrated that variolation was an effective tool to prevent smallpox, but it had elicited an unexpected violent community reaction. In the 300 years between 1721 and 2021, some things apparently have not changed. Consider the violence of the 2020 armed invasion of the Michigan state house that followed an anti-mask demonstration. Two of the invaders were later accused of plotting to murder Michigan Governor Whitmer. Going from firebombing to planning a murder is not a sign of progress.

The 1721 debate over inoculation pitted rich vs poor, uneducated vs educated, with the clergy somehow getting involved in all sides of the issue. This line up has not changed much in 300 years, and the debate over the Covid 19 Epidemic featured a similar cast of characters. The cultural descendants of the 1721 dissenters remain alive and well today.

Modern public health issues continue to be contentious, including the safety of the measles vaccine, birth control, fluoridation of water, and mask-wearing during Covid 19. It is still debated which authority should regulate these issues—the secular, the clerical, or neither. Anti-authoritarianism continues to run deep in American culture. That sentiment continues to conflict with the need to protect the public health during an epidemic. How much of a sacrifice of one's personal liberty is it to put on a mask?

For centuries, American constitutional law granted state governments broad public health powers. In the famous 1824 case of Gibbons v. Ogden, Chief Justice John Marshall defended the "acknowledged power of a State to provide for the health of its citizens." States, he explained, were empowered to enact "inspection laws, quarantine laws" and "health laws of every description."

Houses of worship are places where singing, praying, and chanting occur, and become excellent places to spread virus via respiratory and airborne droplets. That made houses of worship especially good places to spread an epidemic. Because of the threat of spreading Covid, New York Governor Cuomo limited attendance at places of worship.

In the November 25, 2020 decision in Roman Catholic Diocese of Brooklyn v. Cuomo, the current US Supreme Court justices negated that decision. [17] Disregarding the ongoing pandemic that was killing hundreds of American every day, the justices stated that freedom of religion could not be limited.[18] That decision represents one of the failures of public health enforcement that led to the deaths of one million Americans from Covid 19. This gave the US one of the highest death rates from Covid 19 in the Western world.

All this history sets the scene for the main story of smallpox and the American Revolution. In 1775, George Washington (GW) took command of the Continental Army to find that his army faced two dangerous enemies; the inoculated professional British Army, and a dangerous smallpox epidemic that was out of control. The Revolution was in great peril, but against great odds Washington was able to control events, and to secure victory.

1B. SMALLPOX and the American Revolution.

The combat of the American Revolution and the transcontinental smallpox epidemic both began in 1775 and ended in 1782. From the Siege of Boston to the Siege of Yorktown, smallpox played a critical role.

The **first** of several epic events that began in 1775 in British North America was Pox Americana, the continental small pox epidemic of 1775.[1] Smallpox would go on to kill 130,000 people over seven years, a considerable death toll since the thirteen British colonies had a European population of about 2.5 million. Not all the deaths were among British colonials. Black Americans and Native Americans were also affected. (Afro-Americans were counted, Native Americans were not)

The **next** event of 1775 was the American Revolution that began in earnest, with continuing armed conflict between the British and the Continental armies that lasted until 1782. The bloodiest battle of the war for the British officer corps was fought on June 17, 1775, at Bunker Hill where over 100 British officers were killed or wounded in one afternoon. That would be about 10 to 20 percent of their total wartime casualties. That had a chilling and lasting effect on the British officer corps, as they would be hesitant in the future to attack fortified positions. The British casualties at Bunker Hill also foreshadowed a long and violent conflict.

The **third** event took place on July 1, 1775, as George Washington assumed command of the Continental Army at the Common in Cambridge, Massachusetts. This was the beginning of a national army, headquartered in Massachusetts, and led by a Virginian, George Washington who took his orders from the Continental Congress located in Philadelphia.

The Smallpox Epidemic of 1775 was worsened by the armed combat of the Revolution. The co-mingling of military and civilians helped propagate the epidemic. As large numbers of infected soldiers were on the move, they spread the disease. Conversely, soldiers who had no immunity to smallpox marched into an epidemic area and became infected themselves.

Proximity to an infected person was a key factor in transmission, and 18th-century battlefields were crowded and became a site for the spread of smallpox. Military camps, hospitals, prisons and especially prison ships were also crowded and became centers of infection. Wounded soldiers were susceptible to disease. Combat destroyed crops and places of shelter, and that also worsened the outlook for sick soldiers and civilians.

**Opening Day Line-Up American Revolution:
Major Players Immunity to Smallpox,**

- Smallpox survivors: Immune
- British Army: Mostly immune
- Inoculated recruits: Immune but temporarily infectious
- Africans: Arrivals from Africa had some acquired immunity
- Afro-Americans: May have had some herd immunity by living among Africans
- Continental Army: No immunity before 1777, immune after 1777
- State militias: Almost no immunity
- Colonial Europeans: Little immunity because of opposition to inoculation
- Native Americans: Almost no immunity

IN 1775 THE British army was well immunized and had a plan for quarantining all recruits and any soldiers who became ill with smallpox. The Continental Army had no such plan.

The British had an immense military advantage in 1775, taking the field with a mostly smallpox-immune army during the continental smallpox epidemic. They were professional soldiers, mostly inoculated, relatively healthy, and their military mobility was not limited by disease.

In comparison the Continentals had almost no training, were not inoculated, had many soldiers becoming ill with smallpox, and as a result had greatly reduced mobility. The Continental Army could not enter towns where smallpox was raging and, conversely, the army was not allowed into healthy towns.

The final major event of 1775 was the Continental Army's invasion of Canada. Smallpox was killing more Continental soldiers than were the British. This was highlighted by the retreat from Quebec. After initial success at Montreal, the Continentals were badly defeated at Quebec on New Year's Eve, 1775. At Quebec, smallpox was used by the British as a military weapon. They sent infected deserters, prisoners, slaves, and contaminated supplies into the American camp for the purpose of infecting them, and they were quite successful.

During the retreat from Quebec, almost all the Continentals became ill with smallpox. Because they were being pursued by the British, they could not pause to nurse the sick. A special ordeal for the Americans was walking on their very painful smallpox infected feet. Any semblance of quarantine had disappeared in the drive to escape the British.

"Men in the full throes of smallpox struggled through knee-deep snow alongside men who had never had the disease, while others unaware they were incubating smallpox, mingled with healthy troops." This was a death march in the very sense of the word. About one third of the American troops on the march died from smallpox.[2] The invasion of Canada and defeat at Quebec had major consequences for the American Revolution.

Although Canada remained British, the British invasion of

New York state was delayed for a year, since the invasion upset the British timetable for attack. The British could never recover from the delay, and their New York Plan ended with their defeat at Saratoga 1777.

Smallpox continued to decimate the Continental Army after Quebec, especially among recruits. Not surprisingly, potential recruits were staying away for fear of contracting smallpox. When Washington learned that his wife, Martha, recently underwent successful inoculation, he reconsidered his opposition to variolation for the Army.

Washington began to realize that he had two enemies: the British military and the smallpox epidemic. Each of them could destroy his army and end the Revolution. And so, he needed to deal with each of them with a coordinated plan of action.

This was the extraordinary challenge for Washington, who was still based in Cambridge, Massachusetts in the winter of 1775-6. The British Army occupied the city of Boston, Massachusetts, and was supported by a large British fleet anchored in Boston Harbor. The Continental Army was encamped to the west, north, and south of Boston, controlling the coastline and the countryside, and effectively blocking the British Army within the city. A smallpox epidemic in Boston and the surrounding area was killing Continental soldiers, immobilizing the army, and undermining recruitment.

Washington had three immediate goals: control the smallpox epidemic; keep the army intact; and get the British to leave Boston. There were three available weapons to fight smallpox: quarantine, isolation, and variolation and he would employ them all.[3]

The smallpox epidemic within the city of Boston was addressed by *quarantine*. Boston was a virtual island in Boston Harbor, connected to the mainland by Boston Neck, an isthmus only 120 feet wide. By maintaining a blockade at the Neck, Washington quite readily imposed a quarantine of Boston. Hardly anything moved in or out of Boston by land.

When any Continental soldier contracted smallpox, they were placed in *isolation*. Since the Continental Army controlled much of the interior of Massachusetts, GW removed sick troops from the frontlines, sending them miles away to isolation hospitals in Cambridge and Salem. This was cutting edge public health policy for 1775.

From 1775 to 1783, Washington made rules for quarantine, isolation, and variolation for the Continental Army. These were not requests, nor recommendations; these were military commands. With the nation's survival hanging in the balance, most patriots had no problems following Washington's commands.

GW's troops needed to be variolated as soon as possible, but it needed to be done in secret and away from the battlefront. Recently variolated troops became sick and unable to defend themselves. The British and the Continentals at Boston were quite close and implementing variolation in secret was virtually impossible. The close proximity of the two armies also made it likely there would eventually be combat. Washington could not go on the military offensive. His troops were too sick to attack the healthier British Amy, and he had no means of attacking the British Navy.

The British in Boston were surrounded by and blocked by the Continental Army, who maintained a ring of well-fortified positions around Boston Harbor. The British were loath to make a frontal assault on any of these Continental positions. They were too cautious and feared a repeat of the Bunker Hill blood bath. The status quo was a stalemate, which was untenable and very dangerous.

GW needed a quick victory at Boston, but that seemed unlikely. These were desperate times and required desperate measures. Washington had to think out of the box. In July 1775, the Continentals captured Fort Ticonderoga in New York state along with fifty-nine one-ton artillery pieces. Colonel Henry Knox told Washington that he had a way to get that artillery to Boston. Washington listened to the plan and authorized it.

In January 1776, Knox went to Ticonderoga and retrieved the cannon. After a brief trip by boat across Lake George, each gun was placed on a sled and hitched up to a team of oxen. Knox and the oxen and their teamsters and fifty-nine artillery guns on sleds trekked 300 miles along the frozen countryside of New England, reaching Boston six weeks later.

They only lost a single gun along the way, although they crossed Lake George and at least six rivers, (Mohawk, Hudson, Housatonic, Westfield, Connecticut, Charles) and several lakes and streams on their trip to Boston. The guns were taken to Dorchester Heights, the highest point on the perimeter of Boston Harbor. Because of the threat of bombardment from these guns, the British Navy was forced to evacuate Boston Harbor on March 17, 1776. Absent the fleet, the British Army was forced to evacuate Boston, along with most of the Massachusetts Loyalists leaders. March 17 is now celebrated as a public holiday in Boston, Evacuation Day. Happily, it coincides with St. Patrick's Day and is a day of great celebration for the Irish-American citizens of Boston, Massachusetts.

In a complex series of maneuvers, made possible by coordination of military and public health policy, Washington had liberated Boston and forced the British army and navy to abandon the city and the harbor. Over 1,100 Loyalists, including most of the Loyalist leaders, left along with the British. A critical group of opponents left the political and military battlefields, never to return. However, most of the Loyalists were ordinary folk.[4] They were the vanguard for the 80,000 Loyalists who left the United States during and after the war.

All of this was accomplished with hardly a shot fired. The liberation of Boston was won by innovation and intelligence. Washington had controlled the smallpox epidemic in Boston and within his army. He kept his army intact by utilizing quarantine and isolation, by avoiding combat in Boston, and by postponing variolation until the army was in a safer place. The 25-year-old Henry Knox was identified as a capable, innovative and loyal officer. He rose in rank to become the first secretary of war in the Federal Government.

Controlling the smallpox epidemic had been critical, since the infected army was facing a time of great peril. Once the Loyalists left Boston, the balance of power made a very small shift toward the Continentals.

With the British gone from Boston, General Washington turned his attention to New York City, which he correctly assumed would be the target of a British invasion. There was no opportunity to variolate his troops, as Washington was busy moving his army to New York to prepare for combat. Variolation needed to be postponed for a safer time and place, but it remained part of the grand strategy from 1776 to 1777, that focused on keeping the army intact.

After Washington arrived in New York, the full weight of the British Empire came crashing down upon him and his troops. In August 1776, the British invaded New York with a huge amphibious force of over 400 ships and 32,000 men. They easily controlled New York Harbor, which is an archipelago, and that guaranteed their victory. The Continentals were no match for them and were decisively defeated at the Battle of Long Island.[5]

Eventually, after a fighting retreat, Washington led the army in a narrow escape from New York to the relative safety of New Jersey. Even after several decisive defeats around New York City, the Continental Army remained in the field, lived on, ready to fight another day.

Despite their huge military advantage, the healthy, well-trained, smallpox-immune British Army, supported by the British navy, had failed to destroy the sick, untrained Continentals at Bunker Hill, Quebec, or Long Island. They could never quite finish them off.

During the dark days of December 1776, an English immigrant, Thomas Paine wrote the following words: "These are the times that try men's souls. The summer soldier and the sunshine patriot will, in this crisis, shrink from the service of their country; but he that stands by it now, deserves the love and thanks of man and woman."[6]

During COVID 19 in 2021, true patriots have flocked to the colors, got tested, and vaccinated, taught school, drove buses, worked at the grocers, donned facial masks, and worked in the hell of Covid ICUs.

The sunshine patriots cannot be bothered to wear a mask in public. The sunshine patriot will not give up their liberty to get vaccinated, to protect the aged and school children, or to work for the greater good of the community. Public health is a difficult concept for them.

A few months after the Battle of Long Island, spurred on by Thomas Paine's eloquence, the Continentals revived their cause, crossed the Delaware River, and launched a daring surprise attack on the Hessian mercenaries at Trenton, New Jersey on Dec 25, 1776. The revolution continued.

An interesting medical event took place at the Battle of Trenton. On Christmas Night 1776, Dr. John Riker was asleep in his home in Pennington, New Jersey when his barking dogs awakened him. The cause of the commotion was the passing columns of Continental troops en route to Trenton. Dr. Riker spoke with the young lieutenant leading the column and volunteered to join the troops. He added "I'm a doctor, and I may be of help to some poor fellow."[7] So, Dr. Riker joined the column and marched off to Trenton alongside the young officer.

At the ensuing battle of Trenton, the young lieutenant was shot in the left axilla, severing his axillary artery, which was bleeding profusely. That was usually a fatal wound, but since Dr. Riker had marched by the lieutenant's side, he was able to quickly stop the bleeding by either clamping or tying off or compressing the bleeding artery. This was a pretty amazing bit of 18th century field surgery, since vascular surgeons did not officially exist until the appearance of Drs. Guthrie and Carrel (1905 - 1908).[8]

That "poor fellow" treated by Dr. Riker would keep his arm and survive another 55 years because his Continental troops had alarmed Dr. Riker's dogs. The 18-year-old lieutenant, James Monroe, did not die until 1831, the third of the first five presidents to die on July 4. Consider for a moment: How could there be any connection between barking dogs and the Monroe Doctrine?

In 1777, the Continental Army finally found safe refuge in New Jersey. While there, they had enough time and distance from the British to be variolated. That would be the first successfully implemented public health measure in American history.[9]

Afterwards, the Continental Army, now healthy and mobile, could attack and maneuver without consideration of smallpox. The tide was slowly beginning to turn to favor the Continentals. When we judge Washington, recall that his actions preceded all the great innovations noted on our timeline, before Jenner, and Snow and Pasteur, before microbiology or virus or epidemiology were words. There was no NIH, no science advisor. How did he do it?

In 1751, when Washington was 19 years old, he traveled to Barbados, his only trip out of country. He was accompanying his half-brother Lawrence, who was seeking a favorable location for treatment of his tuberculosis. Several days after arriving in Barbados, the brothers heard that one of their Barbados hosts had smallpox in their household, but as men of honor they could not renege on a dinner invitation, that they had already accepted. George went to dinner and about two weeks later he came down with smallpox.[10] He became gravely ill, but survived, and carried the scars of that experience all his life.

He gained useful personal knowledge of the devastating

effects of smallpox and learned first-hand how easily it could be spread. As a smallpox survivor, Washington was now immune to the disease, which was useful for a military commander during a smallpox epidemic.[11]

Washington had some medical training in the early 1760s. He took part in a correspondence course with a British medical school, which sent him books and supplies. He then became physician for his slaves and family.

As the Revolutionary War continued, so did the North American epidemic of smallpox. But with increasing control of smallpox by inoculation and quarantine, the Continental Army was becoming healthier and was no longer immobilized by disease.

The Native American allies of the British, the Iroquois, Creek, and Cherokee continued to contract smallpox as they came into contact with a continuing stream of infected white men, including trappers, traders, settlers moving west, and soldiers on patrol or foraging. There was no variolation for Native Americans. In their weakened state, they were routed and destroyed by the Continental Army.

One example was Sullivan's Campaign against the Iroquois, in 1779 in New York state, which was planned and coordinated by Washington. The Iroquois were destroyed as a military force and were removed from the battlefield. Another British ally joined the New England Loyalists on the sidelines.[12]

Before the victory at Yorktown the Americans continued to lose most large-scale set-piece battles during the war, but their army remained intact and ready to strike.[13]

During their Carolina expedition of 1780-81, British Army efficiency was diminished by widespread Yellow Fever and malaria. The Americans did better with these diseases, perhaps because of their experience in avoiding mosquito-borne diseases or perhaps by some acquired immunity. This was referred to as "seasoning."[14]

Washington sent units of the Continental Army led by his

protege, the Marquis de Lafayette, to harass General Cornwallis, who led the British retreat toward the Virginia coast.

On his way to Yorktown, Cornwallis took the bodies of black British soldiers who had succumbed to smallpox and dumped them all over the Carolina countryside and into the water wells of local residents. This was not how to win over the heart and minds of local residents, the declared purpose of their 1780 Carolina expedition.

The British arrived at Yorktown and Cornwallis decided to fortify the town and await evacuation by the British Navy. For six long and challenging years, Washington had kept his army intact and the Revolution alive. He was waiting for a moment like this. Seize the day!

It had arrived because the British presented a unique opportunity when Cornwallis fortified Yorktown on Chesapeake Bay. He had walked into a trap. This was the long-awaited moment, as Washington began to execute the complex plan to trap the British at Yorktown.

The French fleet in Rhode Island escaped the British blockade. Another French fleet in the West Indies set sail for Chesapeake Bay, and the French Army in Rhode Island marched to Newburgh, New York to join the Continental Army on the Hudson River.

Washington then marched the combined Franco-American army 456 miles from Newburgh, New York to Chesapeake Bay in Maryland. Some troops finished their travels by boat down the Chesapeake, while others marched all the way. The Franco-American forces began to lay siege to the British at Yorktown.

While the entrapment was beginning, Continental troops remaining in the Northeast made diversionary feints towards Manhattan, initially fooling the British into thinking New York City was their target. The critical synchronization of all that complex military movement was only possible with a smallpox-healthy Continental Army, because the epidemic still continued during this time of mass movement of troops.

The movements of the French and British navies during 1781 were complex, but at the end of the day, the French fleet succeeded in keeping the British out of most of Chesapeake Bay. Cornwallis, abandoned by the British Navy due to incompetence and poor communication, was trapped at Yorktown by both land and sea. The British Army was left to fight alone.

This was brilliant strategy by Washington; it required extensive coordination and leadership to move all of the Continental and French forces, including soldiers and sailors.

The victory at Yorktown was preceded by yet another attempt by the British to infect the Continental Army. They expelled 4,500 smallpox-infected black soldiers from Yorktown. These black soldiers were among the 30,000 slaves who had been offered freedom if they fought for the British.

These infected soldiers from Yorktown were ordered to enter Continental lines and cause disease and death. But by then, the Continental Army knew to avoid them and, besides, most of the Continentals had been variolated and were now smallpox immune. These infected black soldiers were left abandoned and unattended by both the British and Americans. They died on the open fields and roads surrounding Yorktown.

Not surprising, 90 percent of black British soldiers in the Revolutionary War died from small pox, as they were never offered variolation. Was that genocide? Only about 3,000 black British soldiers survived and made their way to Canada and freedom after the Revolution.

In October 1781, the Continentals and their French allies stormed the Yorktown embattlements, forcing the British to surrender. This was essentially the last combat of the war. The epidemic of smallpox ended in 1782 and peace talks took place in 1783. Washington's knowledge of smallpox had been critical. In the face of a continental epidemic and the world's greatest military power, he kept his army intact and in the field.

Washington managed the smallpox epidemic that affected every stage of the Revolution. Smallpox was the cause of the death march from Quebec, leading to Washington's decision to variolate the Continental Army. The worst defeat of the war for the Continentals occurred at Charleston, South Carolina in 1780. That was a direct result of a local smallpox outbreak.[15]

Smallpox was the main cause of death in the Continental Army, but Washington eventually was able to find a safe place and time to variolate his army. Washington organized Sullivan's Campaign that militarily destroyed the smallpox-weakened Iroquois.

About 25,000 Continental soldiers died during the Revolutionary War; about half of those deaths were from smallpox. Eleven thousand American soldiers and sailors died under horrendous conditions in the British prison ships in New York harbor. About half of those deaths were from smallpox.

The British threw the bodies of the dead into the harbor. During the 19th century, the bones of these prisoners began to wash up on the shore at the Wallabout Bay section of Brooklyn, which became the site of the Brooklyn Navy Yard. These remains were carried away by local Brooklyn residents and buried in a crypt at Fort Greene Park in Brooklyn. Above the crypt stands the Prison Ship Martyrs Monument, designed by Stanford White. But many prisoners' remains are still in New York Harbor, which is the largest unmarked grave in the US.

THE WALLABOUT MARTYRS, a poem, written in 1888 by one-time Wallabout resident Walt Whitman[16]

> *Greater than memory of Achilles or Ulysses,*
> *More, more by far to thee than tomb of Alexander,*
> *Those cart loads of old charnel ashes, scales and*
>   *splints of moldy bones,*
> *Once living men once resolute courage, aspiration,*
>   *strength,*
> *The stepping stones to thee to-day and here, America.*

Let's close this chapter with a story of a typical American family caught up in the war and the epidemic. In 1780, during the British invasion of South Carolina, three hundred British and Loyalists soldiers leveled much of Waxhaw, South Carolina, near modern day Charlotte, North Carolina, killing more than one hundred American patriots.

Betty Jackson was a widow living in the Waxhaw area with her three sons. After the Waxhaw massacre, her oldest son joined a patriot regiment and died at the Battle of Stono Ferry. After another skirmish near Waxhaw, both of Betty's remaining sons were captured by British troops and taken along with twenty other prisoners to Camden, South Carolina. There, the British placed them into a prison camp with 250 other men without any medicine or beds and only small amounts of bread for food. One of the sons was slashed on his head and hand by a British officer, and both boys became infected with smallpox.

Betty was able to arrange a prisoner transfer that included both of her sons. The younger son walked the forty miles back to Waxhaw, while his mother and his dying older brother rode home on horseback. The older boy succumbed to smallpox two days after reaching home, but the younger son survived.

After the younger son regained his strength, Betty left home and went to care for her nephew and other American soldiers in the prison ships of Charleston Harbor. There she became ill with typhus and passed away in 1781. She was buried in an unmarked grave.

Betty's son was now 14 years old, an orphan, a combat veteran, a survivor of war wounds and smallpox, and an ex-POW. He had lost every member of his family to the war, his mother and both brothers.

"The American Revolution had been one long agony for young Andrew Jackson. He never forgot the price that he had paid to secure Liberty." He had endured great hardship, and he became a hard man, Old Hickory.[17]

He would be the only American president who had been a

prisoner of war, and was the last president to have soldiered in the Revolutionary War. The Jacksons set a high standard for American families who have sacrificed in service of their nation.[18]

Women heroes of the Revolution include:

- **Betty Jackson:** and the other American women who went into POW camps to take care of the Continental soldiers. Her monument, but not her grave, can be found in Lancaster, South Carolina.
- **Support troops:** the thousands of American women who went along with the army acting as, cooks, nurses, laundry workers, etc.
- **The generals' wives:** Martha Washington, Lucy Knox, and Kitty Greene, who accompanied their spouses into the military camps.
- **Combat soldiers:** Mary Hays, Margaret Corbin, Deborah Sampson, Anna Lane, and Betty Zane.
- **Military courier** Sybil Ludington.
- **Anna Strong** and other agents of the Culper spy ring.
- **Mercy Otis Warren** pamphleteer, letter writer, and propagandist.
- **Abigail Adams**, John Adams' political partner and advisor.

At the end of the war, Washington would publicly salute the thousands of "women of the army."

Please use the term Founding Parents when you speak of the men and women who made a nation.

2
FRONTIER MEDICINE HELPS BUILD A NATION

Hundreds of thousands of Americans crossed the Appalachian Mountains, bringing Western civilization along with them. They also carried the spirit of independent thought, of inventiveness, and of discovery. No longer a colony, the US was becoming a unified nation, always on the move.

In 1783, there were five recognized and effective, modern medical treatments:

1. Opiates for pain relief; 1527 re-introduced into the Western world
2. Quinine-like drugs for malaria; 1630 introduced to Western world
3. Smallpox inoculation; 1721 Mather and Montagu and variolation
4. Citrus fruits (vitamin C); 1747 to cure and/or prevent scurvy (James Lind)
5. Digitalis; 1783; Withering published the benefits of digitalis in treating heart failure

In 1796, Edward Jenner's introduction of smallpox vaccine replaced variolation, as it was safer and more effective. These five drugs were the modern medical *pharmacopoeia* going into the nineteenth century.[1]

There were also many herbal remedies, some of them based on the practices of the Native Americans. Their effectiveness was unrecorded and/or unknown.[2] But that doesn't mean that they were not effective. Lucy Meriwether Lewis, the explorer's mother, was a famous herbal practitioner.[3] She traveled throughout Albermarle County, Virginia on horseback, caring for the sick well into her early eighties.

When the American Revolution began in 1775 there was no general anesthesia and no antisepsis. Surgery was limited to wound care and amputation, removal of bladder stones, extraction of cataracts, and use of obstetrical forceps for difficult deliveries. Cesarean section during childbirth was available since at least 1500 C.E. with occasional survival of the mother. Splinting, setting, and realignment of fractured bones were routine.

In 1775, there were seventeen colleges in the US. The oldest were Harvard, founded in 1636, and William and Mary, founded in 1693. There were also two medical schools in the US, University of Pennsylvania founded in 1765 and Columbia University founded in 1767. The education of colonial doctors was not uniform. A few had gone to medical school in Europe, and a few more to Columbia or University of Pennsylvania. Most had been apprentices to established physicians in America and/or Europe before beginning their independent practice.

The Pennsylvania Hospital in Philadelphia was founded in 1751 by Benjamin Franklin and friends and is the oldest continuously operating hospital in the nation. Bellevue Hospital in Manhattan opened in 1736 as an almshouse, but had several iterations over the years, and is now the second oldest hospital.

In 1775, British America was a narrow strip along the Atlantic coast. Expansion west was blocked by the Royal Proclamation of 1763 that forbid settlement beyond the Appalachian Mountains that ran from Maine to Georgia. The mountains themselves were also a formidable physical barrier to settlement.

But that changed in 1775 when Daniel Boone blazed a trail across the Cumberland Gap, which is located near the far south-western tip of Virginia. The trail was wide enough for Conestoga wagons drawn by teams of oxen. These wagons were large enough to carry household goods, tools, farming equipment, small children, and small animals. [4]

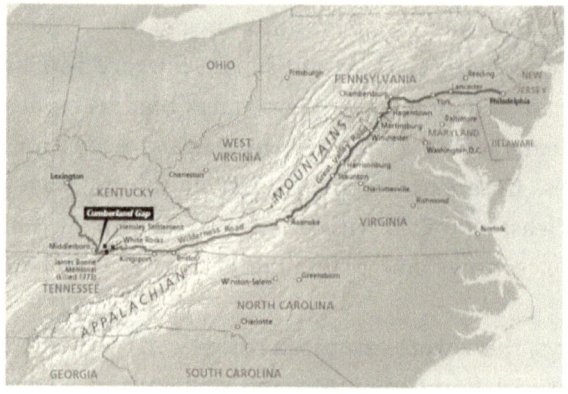

Image 1: The Way West through the Cumberland Gap, blazed opened by Daniel Boone in 1775

Entire families were transported west, as the Appalachians were finally breached. The pioneers ignored the 1763 Proclamation and poured through the Gap, along with their families, music, schools, language, science and medicine. American culture continued to travel west.

From 1775 to 1810, about 300,000 people migrated west through the Gap into what are now Kentucky and Tennessee, including Abraham Lincoln, grandfather of the future president. Many early trans-Appalachian migrants were Revolutionary War veterans, residents of Berks County, Pennsylvania, or part of Boone's large extended family. Some, like Lincoln, were all three.

Another group of settlers were the Scotch-Irish. Exiled from the British Isles because of religious prejudice, they were very poor, and many were shoeless. To defend themselves, they settled in close knit communities in the hollers (creek valleys) of the Appalachians. Isolated from the main stream of settlers, they stayed in place, developing a unique culture that featured their Elizabethan dialogue, their fabulous music, and a skill in the distillation of bourbon and rye whiskeys.[5]

The American people had overcome the first major barrier to the transcontinental settlement of America. As more settlers crossed the Appalachians, they put increasing pressure to expand the western frontier of the US; like helium filling a balloon they expanded the boundaries of the nation. These settlers were strong supporters of unfettered navigation upon the Ohio and Mississippi river systems, access to trading at New Orleans, national roads, and canals. They welcomed new inventions such as railroads, telegraphs, and steamboats along the Mississippi and Ohio rivers.

Doctors accompanied their neighbors, friends, and families, and brought modern 18th century medicine along with them. For example, Transylvania University Medical School, the first one west of the Appalachians, was founded in 1799 only 24 years after Boone had blazed the Cumberland Trail. This evolved to become part of the University of Kentucky Medical School. Other established medical schools west of the Appalachians would include the University of Cincinnati founded 1819, University of Louisville founded 1833, and Ohio State University founded in 1834.

There were also three momentous medical events that happened on the American frontier in the first half of the 19th century. All three exemplified Pasteur's saying that "fortune favors the prepared mind." The United States would no longer be a passive recipient of scientific progress. She was destined to become the world leader in science and medicine. Here are some of the opening moments in that destiny.

EPHRAIM MCDOWELL (1771–1830)

McDowell was born in Rockbridge County, Virginia, into a family of patriots. During the Revolutionary War, his father, Samuel, took part in Nathanael Greene's Carolinas campaign. In 1784, Samuel crossed the Appalachians and moved his family from Virginia to Danville, Kentucky, and became a leader of the movement to separate Kentucky from Virginia.

His son, Ephraim McDowell, spent three years as a medical student studying with Dr. Alexander Humphreys in Staunton, Virginia. From 1793–94, he attended lectures in medicine at the University of Edinburgh, Scotland. He then studied privately with John Bell, also in Edinburgh, one of the fathers of modern surgery. This was excellent medical training in the 1790s.

Dr. McDowell returned to his hometown of Danville, Kentucky in 1795 to begin the practice of medicine. In December 1809, he was called to see 46-year-old Mrs. Jane Todd Crawford in a log cabin in Motley's Glen, Green County, Kentucky. She had not menstruated for ten months and had presented with a large painful mass in her lower abdomen. The local doctors thought she had a prolonged pregnancy.

Mrs. Crawford pleaded for relief from her pain and asked Dr. McDowell to do whatever was necessary. McDowell offered to operate and remove the mass. He told Mrs. Crawford that he had never done this type of operation, but he still felt that he could help her. She agreed, and this may have been the first known instance of a patient giving informed consent.

On Christmas Day, 1809, Mrs. Crawford traveled forty miles on horseback to Danville to have the surgery in the front room of Dr. McDowell's house in Danville Kentucky. After McDowell removed his coat, surgery was performed with the simplest of instruments.

There was no anesthesia and no asepsis. Fortified with some oral opium, Mrs. Crawford apparently sang hymns and recited psalms during surgery. McDowell removed the mass, which was an ovarian cyst weighing twenty-two pounds. The surgery took only 25 minutes, as surgeons of the day were fast and meticulous.[6] Mrs. Crawford, survived, made an uncomplicated recovery, and lived for another thirty-two years.

This was the first successful intra-abdominal operation ever done anywhere in the world.[8] For some perspective, consider that this surgery was only 70 miles and 10 months removed from the birth of Abraham Lincoln in a log cabin in Hodgenville, Kentucky on February 12, 1809. Where did McDowell get the confidence to do such a revolutionary procedure and do it on the frontier? While training in Scotland, McDowell had witnessed the autopsy of a young woman who had a large ovarian tumor. McDowell was well trained and remembered his lessons well.

McDowell's surgery in Danville is a highlight of the theme of this book: the march of medicine along with the march of the American people across the continent. McDowell performed two further operations in 1813 and 1814.

McDowell's experience is an example of the flow of medical information across the Atlantic. Initially it was flowing one way, as Americans went to Europe for training, Edinburgh and Paris being the most frequent destinations. After training they returned to America with their newly acquired knowledge.

McDowell published several of his cases in 1817, and this information made its way to England. Knowledge about abdominal surgery began to flow across the Atlantic from the US. The flow of information now became a two-way street.

WILLIAM BEAUMONT (1785–1853) and Alexis St. Martin (1802–1880)

On June 6, 1822, on Mackinac Island in Michigan, a French-

Canadian voyageur named Alexis St. Martin was accidentally shot in the upper left abdomen. The musket wound was "more than the size of the palm of a man's hand," and affected part of a lung, two ribs, and the stomach. The wound was treated by Dr. William Beaumont, an army doctor who had been trained as an apprentice in Vermont. Beaumont was unsuccessful in his attempts to fully close the hole into the stomach.

One year later, the wound had completely healed except for a large *fistula* on the left side, that went from the surface of the skin into the stomach. This allowed Beaumont to look directly into St. Martin's stomach and observe the gastric juices that were taking part in the digestive process. Looking through the opening of the fistula, Beaumont also saw the large folds of the inner lining of St. Martin's stomach. Beaumont passed a tube through this fistula into the stomach and analyzed the contents.

Prior to this event, gastric digestion was felt to be a mechanical process, associated with churning and grinding of food. Beaumont did chemical analysis of the digestive juices and concluded that much of digestion was a chemical process.[7] Beaumont had put the *internal* into internal medicine.

In mid-April 1833, Beaumont published his observations in a book, *Experiments and Observations on the Gastric Juice and the Physiology of Digestion*. This was probably the beginning of the modern study of human physiology.

WILLIAM MORTON (1819–1868) and Crawford Long (1815–1878); Discovery of Anesthesia.

This is a very controversial history, with several competing claims for the discovery. Many New Englanders are predisposed for parochial reasons to accept that William Morton was the first to use ether anesthesia in 1846 at the Ether Dome at Massachusetts General Hospital. He was first to publish his findings, in the October 1846 *Scientific American*.

One of the other claimants of the discovery of anesthesia

practiced in the foothills of the Appalachians, far from the centers of medicine. He was Dr. Crawford Long, born in 1815 in Georgia. In the fall of 1836, he began his medical education at Transylvania College and after one year, Long transferred to University of Pennsylvania, receiving his medical degree in 1839.

In 1841, Long went to Jefferson, Georgia, in the foothills of the Appalachians, to take over a rural medical practice. During his medical school years, Long had observed traveling showmen who demonstrated the effects of nitrous oxide, or "laughing gas," first synthesized by Joseph Priestley in 1775. The participants in the shows often fell or bumped into things but seemed to feel no pain until the effects of the gas wore off. How do you go from traveling shows to surgical anesthesia?

Observation: Laughing gas dulled the senses
Curiosity: "I wonder if that could be used in surgery?"
Conclusion: Fortune favors the prepared mind (again)

ON MARCH 30, 1842, Long performed the first surgical procedure using ether anesthesia when he removed a tumor from the neck of a young man. This was four years *before* the Ether Dome event. But Long did not publish this episode.

Long performed more surgeries using ether anesthesia over the next several years and began using it in his obstetrical practice. He had made public his use of ether, and this was accepted as fact by his local colleagues. An article about his discovery, along with copies of notarized affidavits of patients and participants, was finally published in the December 1849 issue of *Southern Medical and Surgical Journal*.

That publication was three years *after* the Ether Dome event, and publication. Long did not receive full recognition for his discovery in his lifetime, since he was late in publishing. The consensus seems to be the following: In science credit goes to the person who convinces the world, not the person to whom the idea first occurs.[9]

His life-long friendship with Confederate Vice President Alexander Stephens might have also prejudiced some medical historians. Nevertheless, Crawford Long has an excellent claim of being the first to use ether anesthesia, and he did his work in the backwoods of rural Georgia. With these pioneering doctors, America had burst onto the world stage of scientific medical progress.

THOMAS JEFFERSON'S 1785 proposal to abolish slavery in the new territory north of the Ohio River finally became law in 1787. Most of the 90,000 slaves who crossed the Appalachians stayed south of the Ohio River. They were not allowed to cross the Ohio into free territory made up of the new states of the Northwest Territory: Ohio, Indiana, Illinois, Michigan, and Wisconsin.

In 2021, Thomas Jefferson's statue was removed from New York City Hall.[10] This was a rebuke for his role as a slave holder. This should be balanced against his proposed 1785 ordinance that outlawed slavery in the Northwest Territory. As you do, think of about anyone else, anywhere in the world, who had done such a deed. The Northwest Ordinance would precede the French Declaration of the Rights of Man by four years, and Lincoln's Emancipation Proclamation by seventy-six years.

Kentucky and Tennessee were both south of the Ohio River. Accordingly, they became slave states when they entered the Union in 1792 and 1796 as the 15th and 16th states. Vermont, the 14th state, had preceded them in 1791, and was a free state.

Now the stage was set for the major story of American history prior to 1861. New states were created from the new territories as they became populated with US citizens. This began with the Northwest territories and the Louisiana purchase.

The new states needed to decide on the status of slavery within their borders. This led to a furious political debate and eventually to armed conflict even before 1861. Bloody Kansas, John Brown's raid, and the election of Abraham Lincoln in 1860 made civil war inevitable. That led to another turning point in medical history as the Civil War brought about tremendous medical changes.

3

THE LONG GUN—LEGEND BECOMES FACT

Gun violence in the US is a consequence of the legend of the long rifle, an iconic symbol of American liberty. It was emblematic of the courage and hope of the American settlers, who crossed the mountains and the Plains, and defended the land from rustlers, outlaws, hostile Native Americans, renegades, and wild animals. It was about leading your family through the Cumberland Gap into the Wilderness and providing food for them.

In George Caleb Bingham's painting, "Daniel Boone escorting settlers through the Cumberland Gap," Boone's long gun is prominently displayed in the middle of the canvas and appears as the object closest to the viewer. It is placed to show its significance to the settlers crossing the Gap and going into the wilderness. The legend of the long gun and the legend of winning the West are intertwined.[1]

The legend is also about protecting liberty at Lexington and Concord and at Bunker Hill. The long gun took pride of place in many a pioneer or Western home; set above the fireplace or the front door.

The Second Amendment to the US Constitution states the following:

"A well-regulated militia being necessary to the security of a free state, the right of the people to keep and bear arms shall not be infringed."

Things have changed since the 1780s on the frontier. History gets rewritten to support whatever needs to be changed.[2] In the 21st century, arms have transmogrified from muskets into automatic rifles, and the militia at Lexington Green has become a high school ne'er-do-well who shoots up his school. That has all occurred under the rubric of the pioneer, protecting his family with his long gun.

Gun violence has become a major public health problem, and that has had a major impact on the health of the presidents. The forty-six presidents of the US have had extraordinary exposure to gun violence.

Two of our forty-six presidents, Rutherford Hayes and James Monroe, suffered severe gunshot wounds while serving as military officers in combat.[3] Amazingly, Hayes was wounded by gunshot five times during the Civil War, including a head wound and one severe wound to his left arm. His arm was saved only because of the presence and personal attention of his brother-in-law, an army surgeon.

We have already discussed James Monroe in chapter one. Andrew Jackson suffered gunshot wounds in two separate duels and was also shot at while president. For this discussion, let's exclude the combat wounds. Jackson's dueling wounds will be discussed in another chapter. That leaves six US presidents who have had a gunshot wound in their lifetime, excluding combat and duels. Add five more who were shot at but not hit.[4]

- **Four of the six were killed:** Lincoln, Garfield, McKinley, Kennedy
- **Two were hit but not killed:** Theodore Roosevelt, Reagan

- **Five presidents were shot at, but not hit:** Jackson, Hayes, Franklin Roosevelt, Truman, Ford (twice)

That is a total of 11 of 46 presidents (24 percent) who have been the targets of gun violence, with four successful assassinations. This excludes combat and duels. This is an extraordinary threat to the health of our presidents and to the political stability of the United States. I will review shootings with some brief comments about each of them. With a few exceptions, I will try to avoid naming the assassins; there will be no publicity for killers.

Andrew Jackson, 1835

Just outside the US Capitol, a house painter attempted to shoot Jackson with two pistols, both of which misfired. He was apprehended, but not until Jackson had beaten him with his cane. The gunman was found not guilty by reason of insanity and confined to a mental institution. He was not the last shooter found to be mentally ill.

Abraham Lincoln, 1865

Shot in the head at very close range, dying several hours later without gaining consciousness. The shooter was a supporter of the Confederacy seeking revenge. Those who have considered that to have been the last shot of the Civil War have confused murder for combat.

James Garfield, 1881

Shot in the back upon entering the Baltimore and Potomac train station in Washington DC. He epitomizes famous people who have received poor medical care.

William McKinley, 1901

Shot on the grounds of the "electrical exposition" in Buffalo, New York where surgery was done for one hour without electric lighting, using the fading sunlight of late afternoon for illumination.

Theodore Roosevelt (TR), 1912

Shot while campaigning for president as a candidate of the

Progressive Party. Before a speaking event in Milwaukee, TR had folded his fifty-page speech in two and placed it in the breast pocket of his coat, along with his metal eye case. As he started to speak, he was shot in the chest at close range.

TR checked his lips and mouth and saw no blood. He correctly assumed that the bullet had not entered his lungs. As he began to address the audience, he opened his coat and showed them the bloody shirt he was wearing, and said the following:

"Ladies and gentlemen, I don't know whether you fully understand that I have just been shot, but it takes more than that to kill a Bull Moose."[5] He then went on to speak for nearly an hour. Only after his speech was completed, was he rushed to the hospital.

The 32-caliber bullet had been aimed at Roosevelt's heart, but traveled through the folded copy of his 50-page speech, (essentially a 100-page document) and his eyeglass case, and never reached his heart. It was lodged in his fourth right rib, and failed to mortally wound him. The bullet remained in his rib until the day he died. The shooter suffered from paranoid schizophrenia for which he was hospitalized.

Franklin Roosevelt, 1933

While accompanying president-elect FDR in Miami, the mayor of Chicago, Anton Cermak, was shot and died from his wounds a few days later. The shooter was interfered with by several spectators, including "Mrs. Lillian Cross who hit the assassin's arm with her handbag, and spoiled his aim."[6]

Three other onlookers were shot, but not Roosevelt. Who was the intended target, Cermak or Roosevelt? This remains a matter of debate. Was this a mob hit or a revolutionary act? A major event in US history still remains a mystery. Cermak's apocryphal words remain with us *"I'm glad it was me, not you."*[7]

Harry Truman, Nov 1, 1950

Two Puerto Rican activists attempted to kill Truman at the Blair House, where he was living while the White House was renovated. During the attack, White House Police Officer Leslie Coffelt killed one of the attackers, but was also mortally wounded. This was a politically motivated shooting.

John F. Kennedy, Nov 22, 1963

JFK was assassinated by shots to the head and neck while driving in an open car through the streets of Dallas, Texas. He was shot with a rifle, while all the other presidents were shot with hand guns. He was taken to Parkland Hospital and pronounced dead. His body was removed and flown to Washington DC for an autopsy.

This is one of the most controversial events in US history. Just about any additional statement is conjecture and subject to debate. There is so much more to say, but I will wait until chapter 17. I have also elected not to discuss the 1968 shootings of presidential candidates George Wallace and Robert Kennedy, confining my comments to men who had been president.

Gerald Ford, September 1975

Ford was shot at twice during a three-week interval that September, which in itself is incredible. The first shooter, "Squeakie" Fromme was a member of the Charles Manson group. She was a disorganized person and unfamiliar with guns. She was not a dangerous threat as her gun remained essentially unloaded; there was no round in the chamber. At least, that was her claim at her trial.[8]

The second shooter, Jane Moore, represented a more serious threat, and her attack represented a close call for President Ford. She was included on an FBI watch list but had been cleared before the shooting. She was a gun owner and a competent shooter. Fortunately, her regular gun was seized by the authorities one day prior to the shooting.

She quickly obtained another gun on the morning of the shooting, but lacking familiarity with her new weapon, she narrowly missed with her first shot. This episode demonstrates the wisdom of requiring a waiting period for gun purchases.

Oliver Sipple, a Vietnam veteran and closeted gay man, became the reluctant hero. He was standing close to Moore and saved Ford by hitting her arm and deflecting her second shot.[9] He was outed by the gay community, who were looking for a gay hero. Sipple was not pleased by his newly acquired notoriety. This recalls the adage that "no good deed goes unpunished." Both shooters served long prison terms, and were both recently released.

Ronald Reagan, 1981

Reagan received a dangerous gunshot wound at close range. He survived the shooting due to the outstanding performance by the Secret Service and the excellent care by the emergency response team at the George Washington Hospital. Bystander Alfred Antenucci helped by tackling the assassin as he was shooting.[10]

GUN VIOLENCE REMAINS a major threat to the health and lives of American presidents, since much of Congress remains in thrall to the National Rifle Association (NRA).

4

THE IMPACT OF VIRAL DISEASE UPON AMERICAN HISTORY— FROM THE ATLANTIC TO THE PACIFIC

Victory in the Revolutionary War extended the western border of the US from the Appalachians to the Mississippi River. The successful Haitian revolution in 1803 led directly to the Louisiana Purchase which extended the western borders of the US to the Rockies and beyond. Thomas Jefferson's critical knowledge of Yellow Fever provided him the insight to complete the deal.

4A. THE NEED of the new trans-Appalachian settlers to market their goods was behind the demand for free navigation upon the Ohio and Mississippi river systems. This was the driving force behind US expansion.

After the conclusion of the French and Indian War in America in 1763, King George III had declared all lands west of the Appalachian Divide to be off-limits to colonial settlers. This Royal Proclamation of 1763 closed down colonial expansion westward beyond the Appalachian Mountains.[1]

While negotiating the 1783 Treaty of Paris ending the American Revolution, British Prime Minister Lord Shelburne wanted to entice the new US away from new alliances with Spain and France. He foresaw a new trading partnership between Britain and the US. To promote this new partnership, Britain recognized the independence of the United States and offered them a very favorable peace treaty.

The Peace Treaty recognized the facts on the ground. Americans were settling the land beyond the Appalachians since 1775. BY 1783 there were already tens of thousands of new settlers in the Northwest Territory and Kentucky and Tennessee who depended on free navigation along the Ohio and Mississippi rivers to send their goods to market. There was almost no trade back east across the Appalachians. The pioneers always looked west.

Not only did Great Britain recognize American independence, but they also recognized the new western border of the US to be the Mississippi River, thus voiding the 1763 proclamation. The US was to incorporate the land between the Atlantic and the Mississippi, tripling in size the area of the original thirteen colonies.[2]

The American cause was greatly promoted by the high caliber of their representatives at the peace treaty: John Jay, Benjamin Franklin, and John Adams. They also made sure that the United States maintained their traditional (colonial) fishing rights in the North Atlantic. The Mississippi River then became a contentious border between the US and Spanish Louisiana.

Spain was intermittently interfering with US navigation of the river and restricting the use of New Orleans as a commercial port.

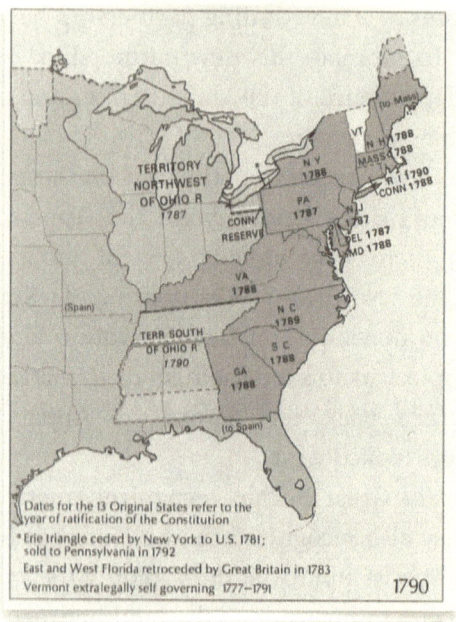

Image 2: The United States in 1790, first major expansion from the Appalachians to the Mississippi

This navigational controversy ended with the Louisiana Purchase of 1803 that expanded the western border of the US from the Mississippi River to the Rocky Mountains. The Mississippi River and New Orleans were now entirely within the United States.

How did the Louisiana Purchase come about? President Thomas Jefferson had intimate experience with another viral epidemic, Yellow Fever (YF) in Philadelphia in 1793. He gained insight into the psychological impact of the terror from that epidemic. That led him to appreciate the French response to the YF outbreak in Haiti.

Yellow Fever is an acute, infectious, viral disease (the Yellow Fever virus) that is transmitted to humans through the bite of an infected Aedes aegypti mosquito. For our discussion, we will only consider the urban transmission cycle of Yellow Fever.

Most people infected with YF virus do not seek medical attention because they have minimal symptoms. About twelve percent of those infected progress to a more serious form of the disease, characterized by *jaundice, hemorrhagic* symptoms, and eventually shock and multi-system organ failure. The case-fatality ratio for severe cases is thirty to sixty percent. YF confers lifelong immunity for survivors.[3]

The impact of YF on American history has been immense.

After the European conquest of America, a new labor force was required to exploit the New World. Native Americans were not going to do this work. Many, if not most of them, had died from smallpox due to previous encounters with Europeans. The survivors avoided slavery by escaping to the nearby wilderness and joining up with their kinsmen.

Indentured servants and bonded laborers from Europe did not do well in the tropics, suffering from the heat, malaria, and YF.

Black Africans should do better in the tropics. Many had the sickling trait of their red blood cells that resisted infection from the malaria parasite. They also tolerated the heat of the tropics better than did others. Many Africans had been variolated and were immune to smallpox.

Many also had immunity to YF acquired in childhood. That immunity gave them added protection to survive the transport to America. African Americans also had acquired some herd immunity to YF by living among the Africans in the Americas. The slavers thought the Africans had the best potential to survive the threats of YF, malaria, smallpox, and heatstroke present in the New World. Accordingly, Black Africans were seen as the prime source of labor and were targeted for enslavement. And so it was that black Africans suffered from the horror and cruelty of the ocean passage and the hundreds of years of subsequent bondage, showing great courage and endurance.

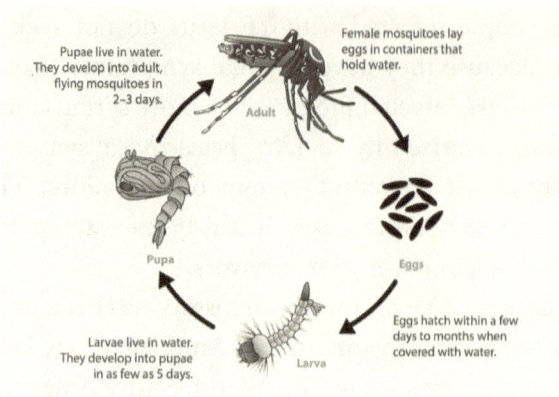

Image 3: Breeding Cycle of Aedes Aegyptii Mosquito, CDC March 5, 2020.

During the long ocean voyage from Africa to the Americas, drinking water for the slaves aboard ship was stored in open buckets. Therein lies a tale.[4] The mosquito vector of YF, Aedes aegypti, prefers to live and breed in man-made containers of water, just like those open buckets.

The mosquitoes came on board the slave ships, breeding in the water buckets, and made their way to the Americas. They couldn't fly from Africa to America, but they were excellent sailors.

This mosquito has a life span of about 1 to 2 months, usually longer than the duration of the ocean voyage, which ranged from 21 to 90 days, and thus was able to survive the ocean passage.

Upon reaching land, female mosquitoes went ashore and found their sources of food, the blood of the Europeans living there. As payment for the meal, the female mosquitos infected those humans with the YF virus. Only the female of the species bites humans, because the male mosquitos, being the docile members of the species, feed only on nectar. This information was unknown until the end of the 19th century.

Many Africans were immune to YF, so although they may have been stung, they were not infected. The slave trade and

Aedes mosquitos and YF went hand in hand, as they traveled together across the Atlantic and through the Caribbean. Because of their relative immunity to YF, the Africans survived the passage and the coastal slave trade, and the full force of the horrors of slavery fell upon them. What a horrible tragedy.[5]

Almost half the slaves died or were killed before they even got on board the slave ships. Add to that, the 20 percent death rate of slaves during the ocean passage. The slave trade was murderous, barbaric, cruel, and indefensible.

The mosquitoes began their trans-Atlantic journey to the American mainland by making a successful landing in Barbados in 1642. Shortly thereafter, cases of Yellow Fever appeared on the island. In the Barbados YF outbreak of 1647 up to 75 percent of patients fell unconscious and never awoke. "The living were hardly able to bury the dead," wrote one survivor. By the 1650s, the virus successfully completed the trans-Atlantic crossing along with its Aedes aegypti carriers by jumping from Barbados to the rest of the Caribbean, Brazil, and then to South and North America.[6]

Yellow Fever was continuously being carried by ships and stowaway insects and would land in Philadelphia in the 1790s. It went on to cripple the city in a massive epidemic in 1793. It also devastated European troops in the Caribbean and Gulf Coast regions, eventually convincing Napoleon to sell French Louisiana to Thomas Jefferson's administration.

IMMUNITY TO YELLOW **Fever (YF)**

- Africans: Many had YF as children, survived and now had lifelong immunity.
- Afro Americans: Protected by some degree of herd immunity, living among African slaves. There may also have been some factor of genetic resistance.

- <u>Native Americans:</u> Had no immunity and no resistance. But Native Americans had very little exposure to YF since they were not involved with the slave trade and didn't congregate in the coastal cities.
- <u>Europeans</u>: Had no immunity and no resistance to YF and bore the brunt of YF.

The French Revolution of 1789 had abolished slavery, but some of the upper classes in the French colony of Haiti objected. This sparked a bloody rebellion in Haiti that was fought along very complicated racial lines. The rebel leadership was largely composed of former *gens de couleur libre* volunteers, free Haitian men of color who had fought alongside Continental troops at the Battle of Savannah in 1779.

4B. JEFFERSON IS eyewitness to the 1793 YF epidemic in Philadelphia, at the time the capital of the US and its biggest city with a population of about 40,000.

Refugees escaping from the fighting in Haiti began to arrive by ship in Philadelphia. They were French colonials, other Europeans, and some American traders. Along with the refugees came their fellow travelers, Aedes mosquitos and YF virus.

The infected mosquitoes arrived onshore and began feeding on American blood. Not surprisingly, an epidemic of YF broke out in Philadelphia during the first week of August 1793. In the face of the epidemic, about half the Philadelphia population fled the city, including Washington, Hamilton, and most of the US government.

The US government was consequently shut down by the exodus of so many of its employees. They later reassembled in Germantown, Pennsylvania and remained there for several months until the epidemic was over. This was the second shutdown of the US government. The first shutdown had occurred on June 17, 1789 when President Washington became gravely ill with an abscess in his thigh.

Thomas Jefferson was the US Secretary of State and was in Philadelphia during the YF epidemic. He did not leave town with the rest of the government but stayed behind to record his observations of the devastation of the epidemic. He never contracted YF during his stay.

But as an eyewitness to history, he saw and heard and felt the full impact of the *terror* caused by the invisible plague of the YF epidemic. Jefferson came to appreciate the terror was the result of the mass dying and suffering, as an apparently invisible force killed 25 percent of the remaining population. Confusion and chaos reigned as an exhausted corps of health care workers tried to keep pace with an inexhaustible flow of patients.

From August until October 1793, about 20,000 residents had remained in the city, 11,000 became ill with YF and 5,000 died. The citizens of Philadelphia reacted with a flight or fight response, and half the population left town. The enemy was invisible, and flight seemed to be the only way to survive.[7]

Hundreds if not thousands of Afro-Africans volunteered to help, as did most of the physicians and civic leaders. Dr. Benjamin Rush, a signer of the Declaration of Independence, worked day and night caring for sick patients, including performing a lot of useless bloodletting. His dedication to duty, in the face of great threat to himself, is a bright moment in American history.

Free black men and women did much of the dirty work, digging graves, picking up and burying bodies, providing bedside care for sick patients. Despite the erroneous belief that free black Americans could not contract the disease, about 240 of them died of the fever. They were probably born in America and did not have YF as children, and thus had no acquired immunity to YF.[8] Only Africans had acquired immunity to YF.

Any herd immunity possessed by Afro-Americans occurred only when they were physically present among black Africans. This information was unknown in 1793.

The similarities are striking between Philadelphia 1793 and New York City during Covid 2020. Again Black Americans did much of the dirty, dangerous and exhausting work of transporting sick patients, cleaning up sick patients' rooms, repositioning Covid patients, and moving bodies to the morgue. Some things never change. Black Americans rarely get the credit they deserve.

Jefferson finally left Philadelphia on September 17, 1793, since most of his staff had already left. The insight that he gained in Philadelphia served him well during his presidency, when he accurately anticipated the French reaction to the YF epidemic on Haiti. Terror! Escape!

By the middle of October 1793, the mosquitoes began to die from the colder weather and the YF epidemic abated, then disappeared. The Philadelphia city fathers' long-term response to the epidemic was to do the right thing for the wrong reason. They did not know of the association of YF with mosquitos and thought that YF was due to poor sanitation and a fouled water supply. Accordingly, attempts were made to improve the city's sanitary conditions.

The biggest improvement was the construction of Philadelphia's waterworks, the first public water system in the US. It was designed by Benjamin Latrobe, whose later works included the US Capitol in Washington DC. As you might predict, YF continued in Philadelphia, but there was less water borne diseases such as cholera and typhoid, and the streets were much cleaner. Ironically, Latrobe died of YF in 1820 while in New Orleans, designing their water works.

4C. YF epidemic on Haiti in 1802-1803, led to the Louisiana Purchase by the US. Thomas Jefferson, the Philadelphia eyewitness of 1793, was the president in 1803.

Manifest Destiny was a phrase coined in 1845 to highlight a doctrine that the United States had a divine right to expand its dominion and spread democracy and capitalism across the entire North American continent. The continued territorial expansion of the boundaries of the United States westward to the Pacific was said to be inevitable. At the heart of Manifest Destiny was the pervasive belief that Americans enjoyed cultural and racial superiority over Native Americans, Mexicans, and Afro-Americans.

However, US expansion across the continent was not preordained nor was it inevitable. It came about by the conscious acts of American politicians such as John Adams, Thomas Jefferson, and James Polk who took advantage of opportunities that presented themselves.

The US purchase of Louisiana in 1803 was facilitated by the onset of an epidemic of Yellow Fever in Haiti that destroyed Napoleon's army. President Jefferson understood the significance of those events and capitalized upon that knowledge to facilitate the Louisiana Purchase. The theory of Manifest Destiny is racist nonsense. The divinity did not appear to be involved in any of these real estate transactions.

Louisiana, the land between the Mississippi River and the Rockies plus New Orleans, had changed hands several times prior to the US taking possession in 1803.

- France ruled Louisiana from 1699 to 1762
- France sold it to Spain who ruled from 1762 to 1800
- Spain returned Louisiana to France in 1800
- France sold Louisiana to the US in December, 1803

The reasons for these exchanges were connected to European dynastic politics and intrigue. It's not easy to follow the sequence of events from 1800 to 1803, but Thomas Jefferson did. He was deeply involved in the sale of Louisiana to the US through the actions of his diplomats, Robert Livingstone and James Monroe, and his confidential agent Pierre DuPont.

How did it come to pass that the US purchased all of Louisiana, when the initial interest of the US was only to purchase New Orleans? The vital concern of the US had been free navigation of the Mississippi River which was guaranteed in the 1783 Treaty of Paris between the US and Great Britain. The US needed unfettered use of the Port of New Orleans, but that was not clarified in the 1783 treaty. Spain owned Louisiana and New Orleans, and they controlled navigation on the Mississippi. The US signed a separate treaty with Spain, guaranteeing the US the use of the Port of New Orleans, but the Spanish authorities did not always honor the treaty and continued to impede the transfer of US goods in New Orleans. The US continued to affirm their need for unfettered navigation and free access to New Orleans.

Louisiana and New Orleans were transferred to France in 1800. Why did the French want Louisiana? It was all about the sugar being grown in Haiti, a French possession. Two-thirds of the commercial wealth of France came from the sale of the sugar grown in Haiti. Almost all the arable land in Haiti was being used to grow sugar, with not enough land left to grow food crops.

So, the French took over Louisiana in 1800 to provide a source of food for the Haitian sugar workers. It was more economical to import food from Louisiana than to convert valuable sugar cane land in Haiti that was generating huge profits.

Still searching for unfettered trade along the Mississippi River, the Jefferson administration in 1801 sought to buy New Orleans from France. The US wanted guarantees for free navigation for the Ohio and the Mississippi river systems.

Meanwhile, the uprising in Haiti had exploded into an orgy

of violence. In order to suppress the rebellion, Napoleon sent an army of 40,000 French troops in February 1802, led by his brother-in-law, Charles Leclerc. That same year an epidemic of Yellow Fever re-emerged in Haiti and killed General Leclerc and most of his force. This decimated French army then suffered a military defeat at the Battle of Vertières in 1803.

The rebellion in Haiti had become very costly to France in men and money. After this huge loss of French soldiers, Napoleon decided that Haiti had to be abandoned. Napoleon was facing renewed war with Great Britain and could not spare any more troops to defend Haiti. He was ready to cut his losses and grant independence to Haiti.

After losing control of Haiti, the French had no reason for keeping their Louisiana breadbasket, and Napoleon was ready to sell. On January 1, 1804, Haiti declared its independence and became the second republic in the New World.

President Jefferson played a major role in interpreting the events of 1803 to facilitate the Louisiana Purchase. He was well positioned to take advantage of the situation.

Jefferson, the YF eyewitness of 1793, became president in 1803. He had been US ambassador to France (1785-1789) and US Secretary of State (1790-1793) and was no longer diplomatically naive. He now had experience dealing with the intrigues of European diplomacy. He also had an ace up his sleeve, Pierre DuPont, who participated in the back-channel diplomacy between France and the US, and helped broker the deal.

Jefferson was the living thread that connected Philadelphia 1793, Haiti 1802-03, and Louisiana 1803. He capitalized on his knowledge of the impact of the terror of the 1793 YF Philadelphia epidemic, and he anticipated a similar French response to the terror of 1803. *Escape from the terror!*

The following is a brief outline of what was a complex and detailed land sale. Initially, the US only wanted to buy New Orleans and had not expressed any interest in owning Louisiana. Why did the United States buy Louisiana with money they had to obtain on credit? Jefferson was a strict constructionist, and buying new land was not in the Constitution. But several aspects of the purchase helped Jefferson overcome his initial political bias.

In the first place, in 1803 it was a buyer's market as France was leaving Haiti under duress and had no further use for Louisiana. Jefferson was aware of the unique opportunity that was presenting itself.

The dynamics of the real estate deal had created the package of New Orleans plus Louisiana, and it became the only deal on the table. Pierre DuPont, Jefferson's confidential agent, was a supporter of the package deal and helped move it along, as would any good realtor.

Jefferson, via his agents in France, took the deal, knowing it could be withdrawn at any time. Secret treaties and threats of retrocession (return of the land to Spain) were a constant concern.

Jefferson had also been troubled by the presence of French troops in Louisiana. The treaty would prevent that from recurring. In 1803, James Monroe was a US diplomat in Paris. When he was president in 1823, he expanded that sentiment into the Monroe Doctrine, which prohibited further European exploitation in the New World.

France wanted the purchase to go through because they wanted the extra money obtained from selling more land. They had no need to hold on to Louisiana.

The US borrowed the money from the Baring Bank of Great Britain, and that began a complicated process that ended with France using its proceeds of the sale to buy weapons for further European adventures, including an invasion of England. The financing of the purchase involved a tortuous schedule of payments, but at the end of the day Napoleon and Jefferson accepted it. The final cost for the total package was only $15 million dollars, of which $3.75 million dollars was used by France to repay debt that it owed to Americans.[9]

International financing through large banks became an integral part of nineteenth century diplomacy. Baring's Bank lent the money, consulted both the US and the French governments, made a profit on every facet of the payment process, and gained prestige and clout in the North American financial market place. They also took an active role in making the deal happen. This was an opportunity to expand their business in North America.

For France the package deal meant extra money to finance further military adventures in Europe. For the British, despite the threat of money going to buy French arms, the purchase would achieve one of their major goals, removal of French forces from North America. For the US, the package was the way to get their real prize, New Orleans.

The US purchase of Louisiana had been very complex, but for a brief moment, the stars became aligned. The package deal joined together the interests of the US, Great Britain, and France. The activist involvement of Pierre DuPont and Baring's Bank cemented the deal. The alliance of all these forces and personalities, drove the deal to completion, the largest financial transaction in history at the time.

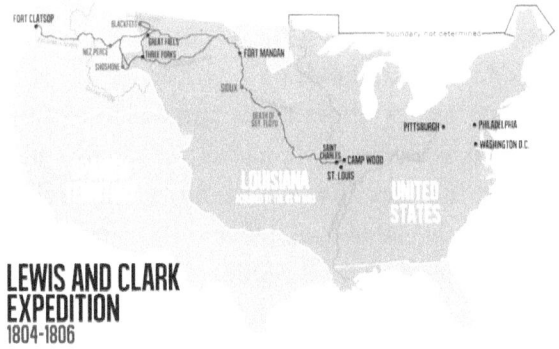

Image 4: Louisiana Purchase 1803, the US expands from the Atlantic to the Rocky Mountains

THE MISSISSIPPI RIVER was now totally within the boundaries of the United States and navigation from the interior of the US to New Orleans was secured. Louisiana was to be an unexpected bonus, a political prize, and an opportunity to double the size of the US.

In 1797, Jefferson became president of the American Philosophical Society, founded in 1743 by Benjamin Franklin and others to promote science and the humanities. It is quite extraordinary that two of our nation's founding parents were first rate scientists. Franklin and Jefferson had made a fantastic gift to the new republic, their love of science, which soon became an indelible part of the American culture.[10]

Jefferson was the major advocate for the growth and development of modern science in the late 18th and early 19th century America. No other US president has been a scientist. He was a competent botanist, and an inventor of several mechanical devices. He had a wide range of interests, including paleontology, meteorology, archeology, cartography, and architecture (he designed his home, Monticello, and the University of Virginia). Jefferson corresponded with the leading international scientists of his time, such as Joseph Priestly, Edward Jenner, Benjamin Rush, Robert Fulton, Eli Whitney, and Alexander von Humboldt.

Jefferson's curiosity about Louisiana was one of the driving forces behind the purchase. He had the advantage of observing events through the eyes of a scientist and could project beyond the details of a real estate deal. Jefferson the scientist, the polymath interested in almost everything, hoped to gain considerable scientific discovery from Lewis and Clark's expedition to the Pacific.

The Lewis and Clark expedition was Jefferson's idea. Its purpose was to catalog the flora and fauna of Louisiana and to map the geography of the area. Was there a path to the Pacific

Ocean? How high were the mountains.? Did the Missouri River reach the Pacific Ocean? What new species of birds and plants and mammals were to be found in Louisiana? Who were the Native Americans? How did they live, what did they eat? How did they get about? What language did they speak? Would they get on with Americans?

Jefferson had impeccable scientific credentials, but he was not going on the expedition. He chose Meriwether Lewis to lead the expedition, and Lewis was being prepared to serve as Jefferson's eyes and ears. Accordingly, Jefferson arranged a unique graduate course in exploratory science for him.

Lewis spent several months studying medicinal cures with Dr. Benjamin Rush. There were additional courses in cartography, and animal and plant identification. Andrew Ellicott, an astronomer, instructed Lewis in the use of the sextant and other navigational instruments. Lewis also learned how to preserve plant and animal specimens, and how to search for fossils. He also spent months with Jefferson at the library at Monticello, undertaking a tutorial on maps and geography. Lewis became a member of American Philosophical Society in 1802.

At the end of the day, Jefferson's scientific curiosity sent an American military expedition to the Pacific Ocean, and America became a new and different nation. In only twenty years, from 1783 to 1803, the United States expanded from the Appalachians to the Rockies, increasing in area six-fold.

Daniel Boone's friends and relatives crossing the Cumberland Gap in 1775 had started a continuous stream of pioneers that now continued on to the Rocky Mountains. Still following the call to keep exploring, in 1810 the 76-year-old Daniel Boone allegedly made it as far west as the Yellowstone River. That's a long way from Berks County, Pennsylvania.[11]

In 1801, Edward Jenner sent samples of his smallpox vaccine to Benjamin Waterhouse, Professor at Harvard Medical School. Using Waterhouse's supply, President Jefferson began the first distribution of smallpox vaccine in the US. He vaccinated his family, his slaves and neighbors, and some visiting Plains Indians, some 200 people in all.

Following his presidency, Jefferson founded the University of Virginia in 1819. That included a medical school, making it now the twelfth oldest medical school in the US.

President Kennedy summed it up best at an April 29, 1962, White House dinner honoring American Nobel Prize winners. "I think that this is the most extraordinary collection of talent, of human knowledge, that has ever been gathered together at the White House, with the possible exception of when Thomas Jefferson dined alone."[12]

4D. THERE WERE STILL two more major events for Yellow Fever in US history. Memphis, 1878 displayed the powerful destructive force of an acute viral infection. YF almost annihilated the population of an American city.

This foreshadowed influenza in 1918 Philadelphia and Covid in 2020 New York City. Referring to this as apocalyptic would be appropriate, as 85 percent of the people remaining in Memphis were infected with YF. There was an enormous racial disparity in the outcome. Almost all white Americans were infected, with a case fatality rate of 67 percent.[13]

For black Americans, there was a very different outcome. About 78 percent of them became infected with a case fatality rate of only 8 percent. Virtually all black residents of Memphis had been born in the US, again raising the question of an unknown inherited YF immunity for Afro-Americans. This remains an unsettled issue.[14]

4E. THE CONTROL of YF in Panama will be discussed in Chapter 5.

5

GREAT MEN, GREAT WOMEN, GREAT IDEAS

Modern medical science has long roots dating back to ancient times. One thread of our story begins in ancient times and continues until the mid-nineteenth century.

5A. The ancient Greeks believed that infectious disease came from bad air, which they referred to as miasma, translated as pollution. Another term, malaria, derived from medieval Italian, implicated bad air as the cause of that disease. These theories would be blown away by the giants of the 18th and 19th centuries.[1]

Heroic medicine stated that disease was caused by an imbalance of one of the bodily humors—blood, phlegm, yellow bile, and black bile. That theory was in practice from 400 B.C.E. to about 1860 A.D. It began with the Greeks and spread throughout the Western world. The cardinal therapies were bloodletting, blisters, enemas, laxatives. Many therapies were quite toxic including calomel of mercury and lead. They were also ineffective.[2]

Physicians would attempt to balance the humors by one of several procedures.[3] The first and most frequent and most dramatic was bloodletting. This was done using a small blade, called a lancet, to make a small incision in a forearm vein, draining the blood into a bowl which was then discarded. Bleeding was stopped by a compression bandage

Bloodletting was such a well-established therapy that rules about its use made their way into the Talmud with recommendations and warnings for bloodletting. For example: "He who is bled must first partake of something to eat before going out; for if he does not eat anything, and he meets a corpse, his face will turn green."

A second method was to change the concentration of the body's fluids by giving an enema or by oral administration of a laxative or an emetic. The laxative of choice was calomel of mercury, which was used well into the 19th century.

The third method to balance the humors was by the process of counter-irritation. By causing a local inflammatory process, one could counteract the toxic humors that were present in the patient. Beetle extract was a common counter-irritant.

Another counter-irritant was cupping. The physician took a small cup and inverted it over a candle. As the flame went out the cup was placed on the patient's skin. The partial vacuum in the cup made the skin pull up into the cup. In Yiddish, cups are *bankes*, and many a Jewish immigrant was skilled in their application, including my grandmother, Sarah.

During the 18th and 19th century, mercury was also applied via intra-urethral injections to treat syphilis, giving rise to the cautionary saying, "One night with Venus; a lifetime of Mercury."[4] Sometimes the mercury was given for a lifetime, and sometimes the mercury side effects lasted a lifetime. Mercury toxicity includes kidney failure, disabling neuropathy, and loss of teeth. This routine use of mercury highlights the toxicity of heroic medicine.

The 2,000-year-old heroic theory of medicine (400 BCE to mid-19th century) died hard, but lasted long enough to be inflicted upon presidents Andrew Jackson (1829), William

Henry Harrison (1841), and Zachary Taylor (1850). For several centuries it overlapped with modern medicine. Only cupping continues today. Unlike other forms of heroic therapy, cupping has no significant side effects.

An alternate theory of medicine was evolving in Western Europe, challenging heroic medicine in the 19th century. During the 18th and 19th centuries in Europe, the building blocks of modern medicine were the emerging sciences of chemistry, physics, and biology.

Into this new arena arrived the control of smallpox with the use of variolation and then vaccination. It was then an easy segue from Jefferson to Edward Jenner to Lister and Pasteur and all the giants of the 19th century. The theory of humors as the source of disease should have become history, but it lingered on for decades.

EDWARD JENNER RELIED upon the power of observation. From 1721 until 1796, variolation was the means of preventing smallpox. In 1796 England Edward Jenner introduced vaccination, which was inoculation with cowpox, (vaccinia in Latin).[5] Cow pox is a mild, self-limited, naturally occurring disease of dairy cows caused by the vaccinia virus, and transferred to humans by contact with the infected pustules on the cow's udders. Like others before, Jenner had witnessed cowpox-infected milkmaids and noted this was also a benign self-limited disease in humans. Pustular lesions of the skin lasted only a few days. Jenner also appreciated that these cowpox-infected milkmaids became immune to smallpox. He then did his famous experiment.

A milkmaid, Sarah, was infected with cowpox from her contact with cows. Then, an eight-year-old boy named James was inoculated with pus from one of Sarah's cow pox pustules. In a few days James became sick with cowpox. After several weeks Jenner inoculated James with the scabs of a smallpox patient. James never got smallpox despite multiple attempts to infect him. This experiment was repeated and continued to show that inoculation of cowpox protected the recipient from smallpox.

Within several years vaccination replaced variolation as the primary protection from smallpox and was adopted worldwide. It was more effective and much safer; deaths from vaccination were rare. Since 1978, there have been no cases of smallpox anywhere, except for a lab accident in 1982.

This great boon to mankind rested upon an experiment done on a child who could not provide any sort of informed consent. Millions of lives saved vs. the endangerment of one innocent child. How to choose? There are several unmarked intersections along our highway of history. Innocence is lost at every turn.

Let's review some definitions. Inoculation is the injection of any biological agent. Variolation is the inoculation of a specific agent, variola, which is smallpox virus.

Vaccination is the inoculation with *vaccinia*, the cowpox virus, used in smallpox vaccine.

It sounds counterintuitive, but it bears repeating. Smallpox vaccine is not made from smallpox virus; instead, it's derived from cowpox. It is variolation that contained smallpox virus, but that inoculation is no longer used.

IN FRANCE IN THE 1820s, the school of **Pierre Louis** was preeminent. Louis promoted the numerical method; the idea that new and valid medical knowledge could be derived from aggregated clinical data. In 1836, he conducted one of the first clinical trials.[6] The numerical method of medicine had doctors recording pulse rate, temperature, and respiratory rate, and keeping medical records of these measurements. They also began the practice of the four-part clinical exam which is still used today.

1. *Inspection:* Visual inspection of the patient.
2. *Palpation:* Hands on touching and pressing the flesh .
3. *Percussion* of chest: Tapping fingers on the chest. First described in 1761.
4. *Auscultation of the chest*: Listening for sounds through the stethoscope.

Rene Leannec invented the stethoscope in 1819.[7] He also described the chest sounds, (*rales* and *rhonchi*) that were associated with tuberculosis of the lungs.[8]

Josef Skoda distinguished one stethoscope sound from another. The sounds he heard in a living patient were correlated with the findings he later viewed at that patient's autopsy or surgery. For example, the heart *murmur* he heard in the living patient probably had been caused by the scarred heart valve that he saw at autopsy. He became very accurate with these correlations, and they became the basis for the physical diagnosis of patients.[9] Most of Skoda's findings were published in 1839 and expanded the diagnostic capability of physicians of the mid-19th century.[10]

New medical instruments came into use.
Ophthalmoscope 1851 (views the interior of the eye)
Clinical thermometer 1866 (measures temperature)
Sphygmomanometer 1881 (measures blood pressure)

OLIVER WENDELL HOLMES JR. was a student of the Pierre Louis school in Paris. After two and a half years in France, he returned to the United States, and received his medical degree from Harvard in 1836. His education is another example of how medical information transferred across the Atlantic to the US. Holmes became a leading advocate of the germ theory of infectious disease, publishing "*The Contagiousness of Puerperal Fever*" in 1843.[11] Accordingly, he advocated the use of clean bandages during obstetrical care. Holmes also opined upon the efficacy of early 19th century medical therapy.

"If all the medicine in the world were thrown into the sea, it would be bad for the fish and good for humanity."[12]

Ignace Semmelweis in 1847 demonstrated that *puerperal sepsis* (childbed fever) was transmitted via the dirty hands of the doctors who attended women. Semmelweis made doctors wash their hands with chlorinated lime water before examining pregnant women. He then documented a subsequent reduction in the mortality rate from 18 percent to 2 percent over a period of a year in his obstetrical ward. This supported Holmes's ideas about childbirth fever.

Despite this evidence, his theories were rejected by most of the medical community of Vienna, where he was located. For the sin of non-conformity, he was confined to an insane asylum where he died a few days later. His legacy remains the command to "wash your hands."[13]

Claude Bernard, (1813–1878), the French physiologist, was a champion of an experimental approach based upon the correlation of the functions of the cells with the newly described laws of physics and chemistry. Biology was an extension of physics and chemistry. A major contribution was the idea of the internal milieu of the organism and the constancy of its function to restore and maintain the balance of nature.[14]

Rudolf Virchow, (1821–1902) the great German physician who conceived the idea that disease was due to abnormalities of the cells and organs. The study of these changes was called pathology. The microscope detected abnormalities of the cells, and surgery and autopsy detected gross abnormalities of the organs.

The correlation between pathological findings (i.e., inflammation of liver cells) with clinical findings (yellow jaundice) became the basis of the modern practice of medicine. The clinical-pathological conference (CPC) became one of the major teaching events in medical schools and hospitals. Among Virchow's students were William Welch, William Osler, Robert Koch, and Joseph Lister. European medical science had taken a giant leap forward.[15]

John Snow observed during the 1854 cholera epidemic in London that illness had centered around the Broad Street water pump. Snow believed that there was an infectious agent in the water that was causing cholera. He theorized that the water obtained from the Broad Street pump was the vector for the diarrheal disease around Broad Street.

To test his theory, Snow removed the handle from the Broad St water pump, so that it couldn't be used, and no one had access to that source of water. The local cholera epidemic came to a halt, even though Snow never did identify the infecting organism.

Think of the apparent lack of association between a metallic water pump handle and a watery diarrhea (caused by an invisible unknown agent). This was brilliant detective work by Snow, demonstrating the power of observation and deductive reasoning; water was the vector of cholera.[16]

Early 19th century scientists could describe an infectious disease, they could point to the suspect vector, but they never could see nor could identify or name the infecting agents. A vector is the agent that carries infecting microbes to patients (see below). There is no consistency to the pattern of vectors of transmission. Similar infecting agents could rely upon the same or different vectors, and vice versa. Here are some examples.

The Vectors of Infectious Disease:

Disease:	Vector:
Yellow Fever	Aedes mosquito; Yellow Fever virus
Cholera	water, vibrio organisms
Typhoid fever	food, bacteria
Smallpox	respiratory droplets; virus
Plague	rats and fleas; bacteria
Typhus	lice, rickettsia
Surgical infection	surgeon's dirty hands, coats bacteria
Childbed fever	doctor's dirty hands, bacteria

In 1865, the British surgeon **Dr. Joseph Lister** read a copy of a journal of the French Academy of Science that had published Louis Pasteur's experiments showing microbes caused fermentation of wine. This also was the beginning of a long collaboration with Louis Pasteur, based on the idea that microbes also caused surgical infections.[17]

International distribution of new scientific knowledge was taking place via the scientific journals of the day. In the US, that included the *New England Journal of Medicine*, founded in 1812; in the UK, it included *Lancet* which began publishing in 1823. Another journal of note is the *Journal of the American Medical Association* (JAMA) published in Chicago. Founded in 1883, it is the authoritative, respected voice of the American medical establishment.

Medical information crossing the Atlantic became progressively faster with the advent of the steamship in 1833, the telegraph in 1858, and the wireless in 1901. Much of that transfer of information occurred with the weekly publication of widely read medical journals, which allowed for faster dissemination of information.

To create a larger audience for promotion of antisepsis, Lister published his findings in 1867 in a series of five articles in *Lancet*. Lister recorded that antisepsis technique in the operating room reduced the incidence of post-operative infection.

To prevent infection of surgical patients, and to keep microbes out of the surgical wound, Lister employed his method of antisepsis. He sprayed carbolic acid onto the surgical incision, surgical bandages, surgeon's hands, and onto surgical catgut thread and surgical drains. Lister realized eventually that the infecting microbes were not in the air but were present on the skin and in the wound of the patient, as well as on the hands of the surgeon.[18]

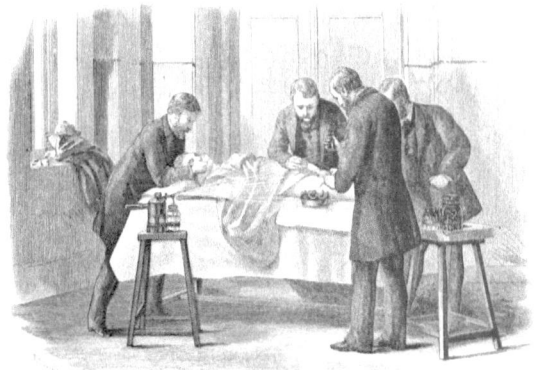

Image 5: Antiseptic Surgery Using Carbolic Acid Spray
(Lister in center holding scissors)

In the 1870 Franco-Prussian War, both the French and the Prussians suffered terrible casualties and both sides appealed to Lister for help. The German surgeon, Richard von Volkmann, became a devotee and used antiseptic techniques to care for the thousands of wounded remaining after the war. There was a dramatic decrease in mortality. It was now an international effort to promote antiseptic surgery in France, Germany, and the UK. These surgical techniques were supported by the continuing experimental evidence of Robert Koch and Louis Pasteur and others.[19]

Between 1865 and 1869, surgical mortality fell from 45 to 15 percent in the Male Accident Ward of the Glasgow Infirmary, Lister's home base. In 1871 Lister examined Queen Victoria and found a large abscess in her armpit. Using carbolic acid antisepsis and chloroform anesthesia, he surgically drained the abscess. The following day the abscess began to re-accumulate, so Lister took some rubber tubing from his carbolic acid sprayer. He then soaked the tubing in carbolic acid and used it to successfully drain any remnants of the abscess. This success greatly increased his prestige.[20]

Young physicians came from all over the world to study with Lister. This cadre of newly-minted surgeons spread the gospel of germ theory of infectious disease. Accordingly, acceptance of germ theory was more prevalent among younger doctors and international physicians.

In 1875, Lister made a triumphal tour of the leading surgical centers in Germany. In 1876, Lister spent two months in the US on tour, giving lectures on the germ theory of infectious disease and the benefits of aseptic techniques. This time around, however, he was received with little enthusiasm except in Boston and New York. The US had been slow to embrace the germ theory of infectious disease. Nevertheless, Lister's tour marked the turning point for US acceptance of the germ theory.

Younger American doctors were more accepting of Lister than were their elders. Several of President Garfield's doctors are known to have heard Lister speak during his American tour in 1876. A few influential US surgeons were converted to Lister's cause, such as William Keen, pioneer neuro-surgeon, William van Buren of New York, who brought hundreds of medical students to watch Lister exhibit the aseptic technique, and Henry Bigelow of Boston and the Massachusetts General Hospital, who led the effort that made that hospital the first in the US to institute antiseptic surgery.[21]

The tide was turning in favor of Lister. The germ theory was now being supported. by leading scientists in the UK, France and Germany, a few influential US doctors, and by younger doctors in the US and the UK. But most US doctors remained unconvinced.

Lister's legacy resides in the surgical principle that *"bacteria never gain entry into the surgical wound."* According to Encyclopedia Britannica, that remains the basis of surgery.[22]

LOUIS PASTEUR WAS the most important medical scientist of the nineteenth century, and he was not a physician. He had a bachelor's and a master's degree in science, and in 1847 received his PhD in science from École Superior in Paris. What follows is a summary of some of his contributions to medical science.[23]

In 1857, he presented experimental evidence for the germ theory of fermentation. A specific microorganism was associated with the fermentation of specific beverages.

In 1863, at the request of the emperor of France, Napoleon III, Pasteur investigated wine contamination and showed it to be caused by several types of bacteria and fungi. To prevent contamination, Pasteur used a simple procedure: he heated the wine to 50–60°C, a process now known universally as *pasteurization*. Today *pasteurization* is seldom used for wines, but it is applied to many foods and beverages, particularly milk.

In 1865, Pasteur was asked to help the French silk industry, which at the time was near ruin as a result of a mysterious disease that attacked the silkworms. After intensive research, he discovered that the diseases were caused by fungus infestation on the mulberry leaves that provided food for the worms. Pasteur developed a method that prevented the contamination of healthy silkworm eggs by the disease-causing micro-organisms. Microbes were not visible to the naked eye and could only be seen on the light microscope.

Both Louis Pasteur and Robert Koch became convinced that microbes caused disease. Koch was a German physician who had spent time studying with Virchow.

In 1876 Koch demonstrated that a specific bacterium,

Bacillus anthracis, caused the human disease anthrax, which causes skin ulcers or pneumonia or diarrhea.

In 1878 Pasteur isolated the microbe, Pasturella, that caused cholera in chickens.

In 1879 Pasteur discovered the benefits of attenuated inoculation, through serendipity. He already knew that older cultures of the Pasturella microbe were less virulent (*attenuated*). These strains of Pasturella had accidentally been injected into experimental chickens. Instead of dying they became immune to repeated injections of increasingly more virulent strains of the bacteria. These chickens then became immune to the naturally occurring disease, chicken cholera.

Because of an experimental mistake, Pasteur discovered the benefits of inoculation using attenuated strains of bacteria, and in the process began the study of clinical immunology.[24] It was for this episode of serendipity that Pasteur gave his famous quote, "In the field of observation, chance favors only the prepared mind."

In 1879 Pasteur demonstrated that the bacteria Streptococcus caused puerperal fever.

In 1879 Pasteur began investigating anthrax. At that time an anthrax epidemic in Europe had killed a large number of sheep and goats; the disease was attacking humans as well. Pasteur confirmed the 1876 isolation of the anthrax bacillus, which Koch had previously announced. Pasteur independently provided definitive experimental evidence that the anthrax bacillus was indeed responsible for the anthrax infection.

In 1881 Pasteur developed a vaccine for anthrax, which used attenuated strains of anthrax. It was widely used and proved to be successful in sheep and cattle.

To honor Jenner and to confuse generations of medical students, future inoculations were all to be named vaccines, even though there were no cows or cowpox virus to be found anywhere in the process. That is how we get to the polio, influenza, and Covid 19 vaccines, among others.[25]

Koch and Pasteur had conclusively demonstrated the germ theory of infectious disease, that microorganisms caused disease and that specific microorganisms caused specific diseases. This theory of disease was the fundamental concept underlying medical infections.

By the 1890s, Lister's antiseptic technique had evolved into asepsis. Carbolic acid was replaced, it was too irritating to surgeon's hands. Hands continued to be washed (but with soap and water.) Surgeons gave up their old surgical coats for clean surgical gowns. Surgical instruments, surgical sheets and all surgical supplies were steam-sterilized, and surgeons started wearing sterilized gowns, rubber gloves and face masks to further reduce the risk of infection. Aseptic surgery was now exclusively performed in hospitals operating rooms, as they were kept much cleaner than homes or offices.

In 1882 Robert Koch discovered and described the tuberculosis bacillus and noted that it caused the disease tuberculosis. He also discovered the method of growing it in pure culture. In 1882 he published his classical work on this bacillus.

In 1883, in Egypt, Koch discovered the vibrio that causes cholera and brought back pure cultures of it to Germany.[26]

In 1884 Koch's postulates were published, which were a method of proof that a certain microbe caused a certain disease. These postulates exemplified the modern scientific method and the search for the truth. The four original criteria are:

1. The microorganism must be found in diseased but not healthy individuals;
2. The microorganism must be cultured from the diseased individual;
3. Inoculation of healthy individual with cultured microorganism must recreate the disease;

4. The microorganism must be re-isolated from the inoculated, diseased individual and matched to the original microorganism.[27]

In 1905 Robert Koch won the Nobel Prize in Medicine for his investigations and discoveries in relation to tuberculosis.[28]

Application of the germ theory was beginning to pay real dividends for the public:

- 1796 Edward Jenner created a safe and effective smallpox vaccine
- 1885 Pasteur's vaccine prevented rabies in humans
- 1891 Filtration of municipal drinking water prevented cholera
- 1895 Successful diphtheria antitoxin was the first cure of an infectious disease
- 1901-1902 Mosquito control prevented Yellow Fever and malaria in Cuba
- 1904-1906 Mosquito control prevented Yellow Fever and malaria in the Panama Canal
- 1910 Successful tetanus antitoxin prevented and treated tetanus
- 1914 the Panama Canal was opened, demonstrating another great benefit of improved public health with the prevention of Yellow Fever in the US Panama Canal Zone. World trade was greatly enhanced, and the US gained enormous military advantage.

5B. (1904-1906) Control of YF made the construction of the Panama Canal possible

Ferdinand de Lesseps, the Frenchman who built the Suez Canal, was unable to build a canal in Panama, abandoning the project in 1889. Several factors caused the French failure. Corruption crippled the process throughout the entire French enterprise. The French attempted to build a sea-level canal and suffice it to say they had neither the resources nor the scientific knowledge required to accomplish this. They failed to account for the unique geography and climate of the Panama isthmus, especially the continental divide mountain range in the middle of the isthmus.[29]

But the most important reason for their failure was their inability to control Yellow Fever. During their project, about 20,000 workers died from disease, mainly YF, including the chief engineer and his family. That was a devastating blow from which the French did not recover. Once again, France abandoned territory in the face of the terror of YF. [31] First Haiti and then Panama!

At this time in history, no one knew how humans acquired YF. Over time it had been shown that other infectious diseases could be transmitted in one of several routes: drinking impure water, eating contaminated food, animal bites, inhalation of infected respiratory droplets, and by direct skin-to-skin contact.

But none of these explained the transmission of YF. In 1879, the Cuban physician Carlos Finlay theorized that YF was transmitted to man by the bite of a mosquito, specifically *Aedes Aegyptii*. That information would lay dormant for about the next twenty years.[30]

In 1898, the US went to war with Spain and occupied Cuba where YF was endemic. In 1901, Dr. Walter Reed and his team demonstrated that Dr. Finlay's theories were correct. YF was indeed transmitted by the bite of the Aedes aegypti mosquito.

Dr. William Gorgas, a US Army physician, put Reed's information to work and began a successful mosquito control campaign in Havana, Cuba, from 1901–1902. The critical piece of required knowledge was knowing the preference of Aedes mosquitoes to breed in man-made containers of water. (See chapter 4A.)

Accordingly, Gorgas eradicated mosquitoes by covering up water cisterns and kicking over any collection of standing water. The mosquitos could not breed and consequently Yellow Fever disappeared from Havana![31]

President Theodore Roosevelt, TR, was instrumental in creating the Panama Canal. He was the godfather for the creation of an independent Panama in 1903. In 1904, the US took control of the Panama Canal Zone with the purpose of building a canal across the isthmus of Panama. Dr. Gorgas was appointed by Teddy Roosevelt as the chief sanitation officer for the Zone, where YF was also rampant. When civilians in the Isthmus Commission wanted Gorgas to be replaced, Roosevelt gave Gorgas his complete support.

This was the critical moment for the building of the canal. TR had understood that in order to build the canal, healthy workers were required. And to ensure that requirement, Gorgas needed to control the Yellow Fever that had been killing them. That required killing the Aedes mosquitos or destroying their breeding sites. This was brilliant reasoning.

What seems obvious now, was incomprehensible at the time. Killing mosquitoes in order to build a canal was original and brilliant thinking. How do you connect mosquitoes to building a canal? Gorgas and TR knew how.[32]

Gorgas repeated his mosquito control campaign that had been so successful in Havana. Once again, he covered water cisterns and kicked over containers of standing water. YF patients were also quarantined. Gorgas used screens for the doors and windows of living quarters and hospitals. The rationale for placing screens around hospital beds was to isolate infected patients. The screens prevented uninfected mosquitoes from feeding upon infected patients.

Gorgas sprayed oil on the roads and ditches to cover standing water and kill the mosquitoes. He paved roads to prevent standing water and eliminated open sewers. In addition, quinine was provided freely to all workers along the construction line at 21 dispensaries. That helped to control malaria. Gorgas' campaign was extraordinarily successful. By

1906, YF disappeared completely from the Canal Zone and, as a bonus, malaria was greatly reduced. The US then had workers who did not become ill from YF and went ahead and built the Panama Canal.

In 1906, TR visited the Canal Zone, becoming the first US president to leave the country while in office. Gorgas had been his man in Panama and without TR's critical and timely support there would have been no control of YF and no US Canal in Panama.[33]

In August 1914, the first ship sailed through the completed Panama Canal. The US succeeded, by building a canal with locks that took advantage of the tropical rain forest climate, the mountains of the Continental divide, and the geography of Panama, and its lakes and rivers. The successful building of the canal was made possible by the application of modern scientific information, *entomology*, epidemiology, geography, climate science, and by eradication of YF in the Panama Canal Zone.[34]

The US was able to control YF in Panama by understanding the life cycle of the Aedes mosquito. That allowed the work force to remain relatively healthy. In 1937, a reasonably safe and effective vaccine against Yellow Fever was created by Max Theiler of the Rockefeller Institute. The vaccine gives lifetime protection to recipients.[35]

6

THE TRANSFER OF PRESIDENTIAL POWER

The peaceful transfer of presidential power is one of the jewels of US democracy. A long relay race is another useful model for the succession of presidents, as one president smoothly hands off the baton of power to his successor. However, that transfer of power has not always been smooth, nor has it been automatic.

THE PRESIDENCY IS a tough and stressful job, and the demands on the health and well-being of the president are extraordinary.

The baton has been dropped and presidents have not always stayed in lane. There have been six close, hotly disputed elections. Nineteen presidents were seriously ill, four of whom died in office. Another seven of those nineteen became incapacitated while in office. Four presidents were assassinated. Teddy Roosevelt and Ronald Reagan survived gunshot wounds to the chest. Five other presidents were shot at, but not hit. Nixon resigned. Clinton, Andrew Johnson, and Trump (twice) underwent trials for impeachment.

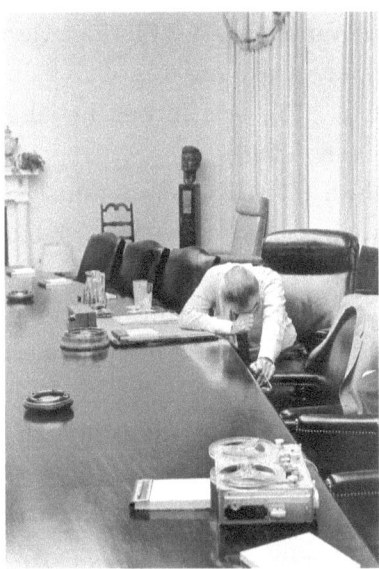

Image 6: President Johnson receiving bad news from Vietnam.

MRS. WILSON USURPED THE PRESIDENCY, and it's still not clear if John Tyler acted correctly in completing the remaining 47 months of Harrison's elected term. To top it off, there was an armed insurrection in 2021 as a mob stormed the Capitol and tried to prevent the counting of the electoral vote. The transition process has withstood all of this and survived.

From the close of the Constitutional Convention on September 17, 1787: "What kind of government have you given us, Dr. Franklin?" Franklin replied, "A republic, if you can keep it."[1]

SEVEN PRESIDENTS WERE INCAPACITATED during their tenure and none of them resigned.[2]

George Washington, 1789, was ill with an abscess on his thigh that was surgically drained. **1790,** he had pneumonia that left him near death for a few days.

James Madison, 1813, incapacitated by malaria for two

weeks during the War of 1812.³ VP Elbridge Gerry had just been stricken with a severe stroke and was of no help.

James Garfield, 1881, was incapacitated for seventy-nine days following his shooting.

Chester Arthur, 1881-1885, was seriously ill from Bright's disease and came close to dying but was not incapacitated.

Woodrow Wilson, 1919, was severely mentally incapacitated for seventeen months following his stroke.

Calvin Coolidge, 1924, was severely depressed and disabled following the death of his son.

Franklin Roosevelt, 1943-1945, was ill with heart failure for over a year, especially during the winter of 1943–44.

These episodes came to imperil the nation because the Constitution specified no relief for the incapacitated president. There was no acting president to relieve Washington or Madison. There was no way to allow FDR or Arthur to take a leave of absence. Most significantly, there was no way to remove Woodrow and Edith Wilson from the White House in 1919.

The ambiguity and uncertainty of Article II, Section 1 of the US Constitution threatened the smooth transitions of the presidency.

In Case of the Removal of the President from Office, or of his Death, Resignation, or Inability to discharge the Powers and Duties of the said Office, the Same shall devolve on the Vice President.[4]

No president has resigned because of illness, or disability, nor has Article II, Section 1 ever been enforced, even though some presidents were unable to discharge their duties and were sick from weeks to years. The clarity of Section 1 of the 25th Amendment (1967) has sent the devolve clause to its demise.

Four presidents died in office, Harrison, Taylor, Harding, and FDR. Four presidents were assassinated by gunshot Lincoln, Garfield, McKinley, and JFK. All eight were succeeded by their vice-presidents, who completed their four-year terms. There was much opposition to John Tyler's interpretation of the Constitution that allowed him to assume full powers for the remaining forty-seven months of Harrison's term of office. But that became the model for the future. The presidential parade had passed over a bumpy road.[5]

Between un-remedied presidential disability, dead presidents, disputed elections, and John Tyler, the smooth handoff between presidents has been threatened or became problematic at least 19 previous times.

1789 Washington/Adams: Washington unresponsive with abscess on his thigh; Adams said and did nothing.

1790 Washington/Adams: Washington was ill with pneumonia; no response from Adams.

1800 Adams/Jefferson: Disputed election with 35 ballots required in House of Representatives.

1813 Madison had malaria and was delirious for two weeks until quinine was given.

1824 JQ Adams/Jackson: Disputed election settled in House of Representatives.

1841 WH Harrison died. John Tyler assumed full powers of presidency, served forty-seven months.

1860 Lincoln's election was a direct cause of the Civil War.

1865 Lincoln Assassinated, shortly after second inauguration, succeeded by Andrew Johnson.

1868 impeachment: if Andrew Johnson was convicted, Senator Ben Wade would become president, but he was widely disliked, and so Johnson escaped conviction by one vote.

1877 Everything about this election was corrupt; it led to eighty-eight years of Jim Crow.

1881 Garfield's agony.

1901 McKinley assassinated; succeeded by Teddy Roosevelt.

1919 Edith Wilson usurped the presidency and the US failed to ratify peace treaty.

1923 Harding died in a hotel room!

1944 FDR heart failure; chaos would have occurred if FDR died before the election.

1963 Jack Kennedy assassinated in Dallas.

1981 Ronald Reagan survived gun-shot wound to the chest.

2000 Gore v Bush: Dispute over hanging chads prompted intervention of the US Supreme Court.

2021 Attack on the Capitol; Insurrection came close to stopping electoral process.

THERE HAVE ALSO BEEN four impeachments, with no convictions. Nevertheless, they are also a threat to the presidential parade. Was Nixon's resignation a threat or a remedy?

There are still many flaws in the US electoral system, and Donald Trump exploited them to attempt to overturn the election of 2020. Federal judges and state election officials held the line and the Union survived. But it was a close call.

7

PARADE OF PRESIDENTS

Prelude to our parade: Recurrent malaria and dysentery were common in the 18th and 19th century, especially in Washington DC. Before 1901, almost all the presidents had recurrent dysentery and/or malaria. In 1901, with the advent of the knowledge of mosquito-borne disease, the swampy Potomac basin was finally drained and cleaned.[1] These diseases no longer were a concern. A bonus was the creation of the magnificent Tidal Basin featuring the Jefferson Memorial and the circle of beautiful cherry tree blossoms. First planted in 1912, they are a gift from the government of Japan.[2]

Our parade of presidents will appear in chronological order. We will refer to our Timeline and note the march of medical progress alongside the presidential parade. Later chapters in the book will be about disability, incompetent medical care and the organized cover-ups that hid the president's health from the public. As we focus upon these themes, we will break away from strict chronological order.

. . .

George Washington 1789-1797: Six weeks after his inauguration on April 30, 1789, in New York City and before the government was organized, Washington developed an abscess on his left thigh. He was quite ill for several weeks prior to surgery and barely functioned. He embodied the government at that point in time, as there was no cabinet and no judiciary. Congress was present but they were just getting organized. Since the only other federal officials were a handful of clerks, the government essentially stopped until he recovered.

Washington was operated upon by the Doctors Bard, father and son, and the abscess was either drained or excised. He had a smooth postoperative improvement and made a full recovery. The government began anew.

In May 1790, GW had another life-threatening illness; this time it was pneumonia. He made a slow but full recovery over several weeks. This was a less critical event, since by that time there was a fully organized and functioning government.

Washington was incapacitated for several weeks during each episode. However, nothing devolved upon Vice President John Adams. He did not assume the presidency during either period of Washington's disability and incapacity. This set the precedent for future VPs.

Vice Presidents Eldridge Gerry, Chester Arthur, Thomas Marshall, Charles Dawes, and Henry Wallace failed to take over from Presidents James Madison, James Garfield, Woodrow Wilson, Calvin Coolidge, and Franklin Roosevelt, when the latter group became incapacitated.

The first two presidents Washington and Adams did not follow the rules of succession as stated in Article II. The first mandated transfer of power should have occurred with Washington's abscess. That transfer never took place. Fortunately, the ratification of the 25th Amendment in 1967 provided a remedy for temporary presidential incapacity, such as undergoing surgery.

John Adams 1797-1801 participated in the first peaceful

transfer of power to a political opponent, Thomas Jefferson. One of the bedrock principles of a republican government, this transfer of power, was severely tested in 1876 and again in 2021. Adams died at age 90 on July 4, 1826, the exact same day as Jefferson died. Compare that with the average life expectancy in the 1820s of about 40 years.[3] President John Adams is the progenitor of the historic Adams family.[4]

Thomas Jefferson 1801-1809: In 1785, while in France, Jefferson fell and fractured his right wrist. Splinting broken bones had been the standard of care since the 16th century. Jefferson's fracture was poorly treated, and he had a crippled right hand for the rest of his life. In 1821, Jefferson fell again, and this time broke his left wrist. Stiffened bandages made with gauze and egg white plasters had been the standard of care since 1812, but they were not used on Jefferson. Once again, he had poor care and was now left with two painful wrists. The irony is this most modern of men received outdated therapy for treating his fractures.[5]

He would be the first president to receive poor medical care. Because of these poorly treated fractures, Jefferson used writing machines which can be seen at his home, Monticello.

James Madison 1809-1817 had epilepsy, apparently the petit mal variety. This did not prevent him from writing the Constitution or serving as secretary of state or as president for two terms. Let's consider him as not being disabled from epilepsy.

But in June 1813 during the War of 1812, President Madison became deathly ill with malaria and was unable to participate in any government functions. The commander-in-chief was out of action. That created quite a problem during wartime. VP Eldridge Gerry was of no help since he recently had suffered a stroke and was quite ill. If Madison died, a disabled VP Gerry was next in line. Could he or would he serve? The Constitution offered no relief for this dilemma. This was a very dangerous time for the new republic.

Who could lead the government during wartime, absent

the president and VP? Finally, after two weeks of fever, Madison received quinine, and after several weeks of therapy he recovered and was able to resume his duties.

James Monroe 1817-1825 died 55 years after receiving a "fatal wound" at the Battle of Trenton, 1776.

John Q. Adams 1825-1829 had a fatal stroke in 1848, while serving as a congressman from Massachusetts..

Andrew Jackson 1829-1837 had multiple severe medical problems that would have incapacitated a less stoic man. Old Hickory was an appropriate nickname, since hickory wood is tough, extremely hard, strong, and durable. Jackson endured severe chronic disease during his time in office.

In 1806, he fought a duel with Charles Dickinson, who shot him in the left chest. The lead bullet was retained in his chest for his lifetime, resulting in *bronchiectasis*, a chronic lung infection that is frequently mistaken for tuberculosis (TB). For 39 years, Jackson suffered from periodic severe left-sided chest pain and frequent episodes of hemoptysis (coughing of blood).

In 1813, Jackson was involved in another gunfight that resulted in a bullet wound in his left shoulder that left him with chronic *osteomyelitis*, an infection of the bone. The retained slug produced severe discomfort during his life until it was surgically excised in 1832. Jackson received the following components of heroic medicine:

1. **Bloodletting**—Jackson had this performed so often that he had his own lancet and bowl and, on several occasions, performed the procedure himself.
2. **Blistering**—in the form of cupping
3. **Use of heavy metals**—Mercury calomel was the most frequent oral laxative, taken orally as a tablet and used as a panacea to treat a whole host of diseases by removing toxins through the stools. Sugar of lead was administered to treat hemoptysis and was also used as a sweetener.

Jackson experienced chronic lead poisoning from the therapeutic use of sugar of lead and from the retained lead bullets in his body. Two samples of Jackson's hair had been taken during his lifetime, one in 1815 and the other in 1839. Both samples were measured for lead in 1999:

- The 1815 sample lead level—130 ppm
- The 1839 sample lead level—44 ppm
- Normal lead level is less than 20 ppm

The 1839 sample had much less lead and was obtained after one of the lead bullets was removed in 1832. These results are good evidence that Jackson had chronic lead poisoning.[6] The *sequelae* of lead poisoning may include anemia, renal failure, *neuropathy*, abdominal pain (lead colic), increased aggressive behavior, infertility, and hypertension. In later years, fluid accumulated in Jackson's lungs and within his *peritoneal* space, a condition called *ascites*. The peritoneal fluid was tapped and drained using a procedure called *paracentesis*, first recorded as being performed in 20 BCE.

Jackson's terminal symptoms of generalized fluid retention may have been due to kidney failure or heart failure, or both. A convincing theory has evolved that both of these conditions were due to *amyloidosis*, a systemic disease associated with chronic infections such as bronchiectasis.[7]

Let's restate Jackson's incredible endurance of:

1. Probable *bronchiectasis* with recurrent severe *hemorrhages* of the lungs and self-administered bloodletting
2. Chronic lead poisoning
3. Chronic *osteomyelitis*
4. Presumptive diagnosis of systemic *amyloidosis* with renal and cardiac failure.

In 1829, Jackson developed swelling of his ankles that progressed to generalized edema, and by 1845 his whole body was swollen with fluid (*anasarca*). During the last several years of his presidency, Jackson was very sick but somehow persevered. Disability was not in his vocabulary.

Jackson suffered from his heroic medical therapy about as much as he did from his diseases. So much of his illness can be attributed to the sequelae of his bullet wounds. No other president suffered from gun violence for as many years as did Jackson.

In 1832, John Calhoun resigned as VP and for the last few months of his first term, a chronically ill Jackson had no VP to succeed him. Jackson's path on the presidential parade was a rocky road, but he completed both of his terms.

Martin Van Buren 1837-1841 was Jackson's second VP from 1833 to 1837. Elected president in 1836, he succeeded Jackson and was the first president born in the United States. He suffered from chronic gouty arthritis, which can be treated with the drug colchicine, introduced into the US by Benjamin Franklin.[8]

William Henry Harrison 1841 left medical school to join the army. At age 68, he was the oldest man elected president until Reagan at age 69, Trump at age 70, and Biden at aged 78.

W. H. Harrison developed apparent *bronchopneumonia* during his first month in office. Recent reviews have suggested salmonella intestinal infection as a likelier diagnosis.[9] He was treated with cupping, ipecac, cathartic, opium, camphor, crude petroleum, and that old standby, Virginia snakeroot, which was ineffective against snake venom and was also *nephrotoxic*.

In the end, Harrison submitted to bloodletting before he died. This was another example of heroic medicine that killed more patients than it cured. Even by 1841 standards, Harrison received bad care. The rumor began that Harrison had been poisoned by John Calhoun so that Harrison's pro-slavery VP John Tyler would become president.

The real culprit had been his food or water contaminated with salmonella. One hundred and seventy-one years later, contaminated food remains a major health problem despite the efforts of the Food and Drug Administration, created in 1906.

John Tyler 1841-1845: Upon the death of W.H. Harrison, Tyler set the precedent for the vice president to assume the presidency of his dead predecessor. Was this the intent of the Constitution? Let's look again at Article II Section 1:

In Case of the Removal of the President from Office, or of his Death, Resignation, or *Inability to discharge the Powers and Duties of the said Office, the Same shall devolve on the Vice President.*

It does not say that the vice president will *assume* the presidency, which would be clear enough. No, it says that the powers and duties of the presidency *shall devolve* on the vice president. Here is the current Merriam Webster Dictionary definition of devolve:

"*to pass (responsibility, power, etc.) from one person or group to another person or group at a lower level of authority.*"

Many of Tyler's opponents wanted him to be only *acting* president. They felt that Tyler's assumption of full power of the presidency was extra-constitutional. Tyler was a Democrat, while the rest of the government were Whigs. In reality, the opposition to Tyler's assumption of power was probably political.

Tyler immediately took the oath of office and assumed the full powers of the presidency, and served the remainder of Harrison's four-year term. So did Vice Presidents Millard Fillmore, Andrew Johnson, Chester Arthur, Teddy Roosevelt, Calvin Coolidge, Harry Truman, and Lyndon Johnson.

Tyler's succession worked well enough after a president died, but there was no remedy for the disability of the president until the 25th Amendment to the Constitution was adopted in 1967.

John Tyler might also be called the *"father of our country"* with fifteen children with his two wives. Although he was born in 1790, two of his grandsons were still alive in 2019. Lyon Tyler, passed away in October 2020, leaving only one grandson, Harrison R. Tyler, still alive as of January 2023 at age 94.[10]

James Polk: 1845-1849: As a young man he had a bladder stone removed by Dr. Ephraim McDowell. As an adult, he suffered from chronic diarrhea and probably malaria.

Zachary Taylor 1849-1850: was a southerner who opposed the expansion of slavery. At the White House, on July 4, 1850, he ate a large number of raw cherries in the afternoon and had another portion later in the evening. He soon developed severe abdominal pain and was treated with opiates with some relief. Dysentery and vomiting occurred, and he was also treated with useless *heroic therapy*, including bloodletting and blisters produced from the extract of the blister beetle. He died five days later, on July 9, 1850. The likely cause of death was a *salmonella enteric* infection.

Unfortunately, Taylor was not allowed to lie in peace due to widespread belief that he, too, was poisoned by pro-slavery southerners. It couldn't be Calhoun this time, as he had died a few months before Taylor.

On June 17, 1991, 141 years postmortem, permission was finally granted to exhume his body to test for evidence of poisoning. Taylor's remains were transported to the Office of Chief Medical Examiner of Kentucky where they underwent extensive testing for poisons. Only trace amounts of arsenic were found with the conclusion of insufficient evidence of poisoning. However, some critics were not satisfied and argued that the arsenic tests were performed incorrectly. They have raised the issue of additional postmortem exams.

Should future presidents have the expectation to lie in peace after death, or are they to be forever at the mercy of the ongoing morbid curiosity of historians?

Millard Fillmore 1850-1853 was the first VP to follow John Tyler's precedent and assumed the full power and authority of the presidency following the death of a sitting president, Zachary Taylor. The rules for the transfer of power had been unofficially changed, and no one seemed to mind.

Franklin Pierce 1853-1857 was the first of three presidents along with Lincoln and Coolidge to become depressed after watching a young son die. For Pierce, the circumstances were horrific. Just before his inauguration, his son died right in front of him during a train accident. This led to the worsening of his alcoholism, which was probably disabling.

Pierce was a depressed, a chronic alcoholic and put in a poor performance, but he managed to finish his term in office. His presidency was a disaster, with his rigid enforcement of the Fugitive Slave Law and his signing of the Kansas-Nebraska Act. Both of these laws propelled the US toward the Civil War. He died from cirrhosis of the liver after leaving office.

James Buchanan 1857-1861 survived a toxic case of dysentery that killed several people at his pre-inaugural party at the National Hotel in Washington.

In 1860, Buchanan's failure to defend the Union almost ended the history of the presidential parade. The southern states were allowed to secede without any interference by the federal government. The secessionist states occupied US forts and seized federal armories. Buchanan did not respond and the survival of the Union was left uncertain.

Abraham Lincoln's 1861-1865 election in 1860 made the Civil War inevitable. This is the most disturbing sentence of the book. The bonds of union were deceptively thin. Nothing had meaning, and all was destroyed in this first modern war. Unarmored men charged into repeating rifle fire. The American Civil War with 680,000 dead, certainly contributed to Lincoln's chronic depression.

Lincoln suffered from significant depression for several years, which he treated with mercury-containing pills until 1861. He displayed many of the clinical features of depression, i.e., persistent melancholic mood, public displays of grief, recurrent thoughts of death and suicide that were exacerbated by the Civil War, the death of his son, Willie, from typhoid in 1862, the "army" of office seekers looking for appointment to a federal job, and the unsuccessful generals who preceded Grant.

Although Lincoln was quite depressed, he was not disabled. He functioned at a high level, successfully prosecuting the Civil War, preserving the Union, selecting General Grant for military command, signing the Emancipation Proclamation; championing the 13th Amendment which ended slavery in the US, writing the Gettysburg Address and the Second Inaugural Address, enrolling blacks into the Union Army, and championing the Homestead Act. This gives testimony to his high level of function despite being depressed.

The Battle of Gettysburg was fought in July of 1863, but the cemetery wasn't dedicated until November. Lincoln went off to Gettysburg, Pennsylvania, to take part in the ceremony. During the November 19 ceremony, Lincoln felt weak and ill during the ceremony and made a very brief speech of only ten sentences and 272 words, and which took about two minutes to deliver. But what a glorious two minutes they were: "...the government of the people, by the people, and for the people shall not perish from the earth."

By the time Lincoln returned to Washington, his weakness had progressed, and he had become feverish. By the fourth day of symptoms, a red rash appeared which developed into scattered blisters by the next day. Dr. Washington van Bibber was called in for consultation and he diagnosed varioloid, a mild case of smallpox. Consider for a moment, the greatest speech in American history composed and delivered while Lincoln was in the second phase of smallpox. Smallpox would be the only disease that stopped Lincoln from performing as president.

By day 19 of the illness, the marks of the rash were still visible. The weakness persisted, preventing Lincoln from returning to work for 25 days before he recovered. The diagnosis of small pox was based on the appearance of a rash, a 29-day illness, and a physician's diagnosis. The last piece of supporting evidence for the diagnosis comes from the experience of Lincoln's valet, William H. Johnson, who accompanied Lincoln to Gettysburg and developed a more typical case of smallpox, dying from it on January 12, 1864. It was a close call for Lincoln and the Union.[11]

Lincoln was the third president (after Washington and Jackson) to have smallpox. The wide spread use of the Jenner vaccine led to a steady decline in the incidence of smallpox, with the last case in the US occurring in 1949.[12]

Abraham Lincoln also had many features of Marfan's Syndrome. He was the tallest president at six foot, four inches. He had very long arms, legs, and fingers, and large hands and feet. Many of his contemporaries felt that he was the strongest man they knew.

The peace of Lincoln's grave has been in jeopardy. In 1876, a plot to rob Lincoln's body and hold it for ransom almost succeeded. In 1992, there was a legal plan to exhume Lincoln's body to test for Marfan's syndrome. That plan was put on hold until better diagnostic tests for Marfan's syndrome became available. Lincoln has no living direct descendants to act as surrogates for DNA testing or to legally protect his remains.[13]

Andrew Johnson 1865-1869 tried to negate the 13th and 14th Amendment and reimpose Negro bondage. His impeachment was a constitutional crisis, placing the Union in danger. He was not an alcoholic, although he was drunk at his inauguration.

Ulysses S. Grant 1869-1877 was an alcoholic, but only as a binge drinker, which occurred during times of rest. He rarely drank when on duty, so he was not disabled during his presidency. During the Civil War his aides carefully watched that he not imbibe while at the front.

He smoked as many as 20 cigars a day, which was the apparent cause of the throat cancer he developed after he left office. Although quite ill, he wrote and completed his autobiography, one of the best ever written by an American. He was assisted in this endeavor by Mark Twain.

Rutherford B. Hayes 1877-1881 was an active and healthy president. He survived five separate gun-shot wounds in the Civil War.

James Garfield. 1881: Nobody provided for executive function of the government during much of the 79 days that Garfield lay in agony with pus draining from his back and face.

Chester Arthur 1881-1885: was a sick man with no VP to replace him. For the three weeks no one was in the line of succession. He had chronic *glomerulonephritis and* came close to death during a trip to Florida. He was the first president to categorically deny his disease.

Grover Cleveland, 1885-1889, 1893-1897: When FDR was five, his father took him to meet President Grover Cleveland. President Cleveland said to him, "My little man, I am making a strange wish for you. It is that you may never be president of the United States."

In 1893 President Cleveland arranged a spectacular cover up of his cancer surgery. Ether anesthesia was used with electrocautery, an explosive combination.

Benjamin Harrison 1889-1893 had no specific diseases noted during his presidency.

William McKinley 1897-1901 was assassinated at a World Exposition that featured the modern marvels of electricity. His surgeons did not utilize the technology that was available on site, i.e., electric lights and X-rays. He died several days post-operatively.

Theodore Roosevelt 1901-1909: had severe asthma for much of his early years that lessened over time. In 1902, a carriage accident in Pittsfield, Massachusetts, led to chronic, recurrent *osteomyelitis* of his legs. In 1914, while going down the *River of Doubt* in Brazil, he almost died from an unknown disease.

He died suddenly at age 60. Sudden death in a 60-year-old

man in 1919 is likely to have been a heart attack. Many studies have been done about the causes of sudden death. All through the 20th century, the number one cause of sudden death was and still is, acute coronary artery disease.[14]

William Howard Taft: 1909-1913: While in the Philippines in 1902, Taft developed *amebic dysentery*, and had amebic *abscess* surgery on three separate occasions.

In order to relieve the stress of the presidency, Taft ate huge amounts of food and weighed 350 pounds during his second year in office. This highlights how stressful it is to be president. He showed all the major signs of the *Pickwickian syndrome,* named for the somnolent fat boy in Charles Dickens' "Pickwick Papers." He was markedly obese and suffered from somnolence sleeping while eating, standing, or talking due to the impaired mechanics of respiration.

Taft lost 106 pounds after leaving the White House. Apparently, he had less stress. He lived until age 77, when he died from heart disease.

Woodrow Wilson: 1913-1921: During his second term in office, he suffered a severe stroke that would change world history. His failure to resign the presidency was a disaster for the nation and the world. He left the political arena and went into seclusion for seventeen months. During this time, his wife, Edith Wilson, along with his secretary, Joseph Tumulty, and his doctor, Cary Grayson, assumed the executive function of the government.

The incidence of stroke in the US has been declining since 1900. Contributing factors include the control of hypertension, smoking cessation, and control of blood lipid levels. Much of this success can be attributed to successful public health campaigns.

Warren Harding: 1921-1923: The circumstances surrounding his death remain as much of a mystery today as they did when he died in 1923. Several of his friends thought he was suicidal at the time of his death.

In 2020, Warren Harding's grandson sought to exhume his grandfather's remains in order to legitimize his own ancestry.[15] Toxicology tests could also be done to answer the allegations that President Harding might have been murdered by poisoning. The courts of Ohio denied the request.

Calvin Coolidge: 1923-1929: In the *Atlantic* issue of December 31, 2003, Jack Beatty reviewed the following book: *The Tormented President: Calvin Coolidge, Death, and Clinical Depression,* by R.E. Gilbert. This biography placed Coolidge's presidency in the context of the deep depression into which he fell following the death of his son.[16] Excerpts from this review appear below.

On June 30, 1924, the president's children, Calvin Jr. and his older brother, John, played several sets of tennis with two White House doctors. The following day Calvin Jr. did not show up for the next match, as he was in bed with a fever. He developed an infected blister on one of his toes. Despite being hospitalized at Walter Reed General Hospital, the infection spread and killed him five days later. Antibiotics were not available in 1924. "Coolidge ceased to function as President after the death of his sixteen-year-old son. Depression had stopped Calvin Coolidge cold."

He displayed the following symptoms of major depression as listed by the American Psychiatric Association. "You may be considered to be suffering from depression, if, for a period of two weeks or more, your mood is depressed and you take little pleasure (anhedonia) in your activities, and you have slowed speech, decreased energy, feelings of worthlessness or guilt, difficulty in concentrating, reluctance to speak at all..."[17]

Before his son's death, the *Boston Globe* wrote that President Coolidge was more communicative than any previous president with the possible exception of Theodore Roosevelt. After his son's death, Coolidge earned the nickname "*Silent Cal.*"

When Coolidge assumed the presidency after Warren Harding, "he enjoyed his position of power. He came to see

Calvin Jr.'s death as a punishment for reveling in the perks and pomp of office."

This man, who had been famous for his diligence, now worked less than four hours a day. After July 1924, he deferred to Congress and declined to use his powers as president. He refused to assist members of his administration in making decisions, and shied away from foreign policy issues. He was fortunate to have Herbert Hoover in his Cabinet, who functioned as an "under-Secretary of Everything" and assisted Coolidge in performing his executive functions.[18]

Lincoln, Pierce, and Coolidge all had significant clinical depression, but Lincoln functioned at a very high level and was not disabled. Pierce's depression was worsened by his alcoholism and he functioned at a mediocre level. Coolidge hardly functioned at all.

Herbert Hoover 1929-1933: was a very healthy adult, dying at age 90. But at age two, he had contracted the croup and was so ill that he was thought to have died. He was laid out with pennies on his eyes. Fortunately, he was resuscitated by his uncle.

Franklin Roosevelt 1933-1945: was paralyzed but not disabled from polio. His rehabilitation is one of the great success stories of the 20th century. FDR was in marked heart failure in February 1945 while at Yalta, placing his own life and the world in great danger.

Harry Truman 1945-1953: In 1894 at age ten, he had *diphtheria* that caused paralysis of his legs for several months. Diphtheria anti-toxin was not available until 1895, a year too late for Truman. He was too weak to walk, so he was wheeled about in a baby carriage.

He made a complete recovery with no residual paralysis. Maybe that is the genesis for his famous "morning constitutional," which was a brisk walk around the block. Harry Truman created his own niche in American history. He was an ordinary man carried along by history to do great things. Truman was a very healthy adult and lived until age 88.

Dwight Eisenhower 1953-1961 had a heart attack during his presidency. Doctors participated in the discussion of his fitness to run for reelection in 1956. This involved them in the electoral process, although they are not mentioned in the Constitution.

John F Kennedy 1961-1963: took part in a massive cover-up of his very complicated medical history. He was assassinated in 1963.

Lyndon Johnson 1963-1969: had clinical coronary disease before and after, but not during his presidency. Johnson was hospitalized for pneumonia and again for cholecystectomy during his presidency and had an uneventful recovery from each. In 1973, he died of a heart attack aged 64, after he was found to have inoperable coronary disease.

In 1965 Medicare was enacted due to the political leadership of Johnson. Almost everyone over the age of 65 now had access to medical care, financially supported by the federal government. Overnight the health and wealth of senior citizens improved enormously. This places Johnson in the very select company of Eisenhower and FDR as presidents who made direct contributions to the health of the nation.

Of interest is the orchestrated political campaign that attacked the mental status of Barry Goldwater, Johnson's 1964 Republican opponent for president. There was much hysteria that Barry Goldwater was a lunatic who would unleash a nuclear Armageddon upon the world.

This was high-lighted in the famous TV advertisement, "The Daisy Ad" that began with a video of a child picking daisies, followed by the audio of a rocket launch count down, then by a video clip of the iconic atomic bomb mushroom cloud. This was a sophisticated high-tech audio-visual slander of Barry Goldwater.

Fact magazine for September–October 1964 published a special issue with every page given over to the feature article titled, "The Unconscious of a Conservative: A Special Issue on the Mind of Barry Goldwater." The highlight of the issue was a survey of 12,000 psychiatrists who were sent the following, "Do you think that Barry Goldwater is psychologically fit to serve as President of the United States?" Of the 2,400 doctors who responded, 1,189 said Goldwater was unfit for office.

"In light of the leading question and the low response rate, it was hard to argue that the survey was useful or even valid—except for political purposes." So said *Psychology Today* in its August 2020 issue. None of the psychiatrists did any sort of physical or mental evaluation of Goldwater. They did not examine him or review any of his medical records. The *Fact* article was a low point in US medical history. Goldwater sued for libel and won, a decision upheld by the US Supreme Court.

This episode led to the "Goldwater rule," issued by the American Psychiatric Association (APA). The first edition of the APA's Principles of Medical Ethics, published in 1973, states that "...a psychiatrist may share with the public his or her expertise about psychiatric issues in general. However, it is unethical for a psychiatrist to offer a professional opinion unless he or she has conducted an examination and has been granted proper ... authorization for such a statement." The Goldwater rule is still in effect.[19]

Nevertheless, during the 2016 presidential campaign, hundreds of psychiatrists publicly offered the opinion that Donald Trump was mentally unfit for office. Once again, they made that opinion without examining the man or his medical records.

Richard Nixon: 1969-1974: Alexander Butterfield, who had been Nixon's aide, once told an audience in San Diego that Nixon was the strangest man that he had ever met. Were Nixon's conversations in 1974 with the portraits in the White House evidence of mental illness? Or were they the one time act of a man facing ruin? How about stories of his erratic behavior after drinking alcohol? In clinical medicine innuendo, second hand stories and speculation do not rise to the level of a firm diagnosis. That pertains to Goldwater and Nixon and now to Trump.

Only one president, Richard Nixon, has sought mental health therapy. He consulted with an internist, Dr. Arnold Hutschnecker, who specialized in psychosomatic medicine. Nixon should be applauded for this and not castigated. His problems with concomitant use of alcohol and tranquilizers are not evidence of mental illness, nor are his visits to Dr. Hutschnecker.

During the 1960 electoral campaign, Nixon developed a *streptococcal* bacterial infection of his left knee joint, a serious disease. He was hospitalized for two weeks and received intravenous antibiotics. Upon discharge from hospital, he tried to make up for lost time and undertook a rigorous whirlwind schedule.

He had lost ten pounds, he was fatigued and stressed. During this time, he participated in the first televised political debate with JFK. Just before the debate he re-injured his left knee when it was struck by his car door. It must have been quite painful.

He lost that first debate because he appeared on TV as what he was: a sick man. In contrast, JFK's campaign was all about appearances, charisma, and vigor. Contrary to the prevailing opinion, members of the debate's radio audience thought Nixon had won [20]

In 1965, Nixon developed venous thrombosis in the left leg after a lengthy trip by airplane. This was the onset of chronic *phlebitis* (inflammation of his veins) of his legs. His treatment was sporadic and his compliance with treatment less than satisfactory.

In June 1974, President Nixon flew to the Middle East while suffering from an episode of acute phlebitis. The chronic recurrent phlebitis of his legs had worsened, and his doctors had advised both rest and hospitalization. He refused and continued his quest for world peace.

Some have wondered what sort of therapy he received on board his airplane. How was that managed? Was there a medical lab on board Air Force One? You might assume that he would receive better care in a hospital.

Pulmonary embolism is a real and constant complication of phlebitis and is often fatal. How would you or could you make that diagnosis on an airplane? How would you treat it on an airplane? It is difficult to follow the thread of Nixon's actions. Was he in a state of denial about impeachment? Was he a heroic champion for the West in his quest for world peace? Or was he suicidal?

He returned to the US from the Middle East and several days later flew to the USSR to meet with Leonid Brezhnev, again traveling with signs of active phlebitis. Imagine that he had a pulmonary embolism on one of those trips. Do you think he would agree to being hospitalized in Minsk or Cairo? These scenarios are worrisome. Can you imagine if Nixon died in a Soviet hospital? Or if VP Ford had to invoke the 25th Amendment while Nixon was in hospital overseas?

Nixon put his life on the line in 1974 with these two airplane trips to the USSR and to the Middle East. Like FDR, his dedication to duty, and sense of service was extraordinary.

On August 9, 1974, Nixon resigned the presidency.[21] Shortly after his resignation on October 26, 1974, he sought medical care because he had a *pulmonary embolism* caused by his chronic phlebitis.[21] Those recent overseas flights were, in fact, of significant risk to him.

He had vascular surgery and a clip was placed on the left external iliac vein above the top of a blood clot. This operation is rarely performed, since most surgeons would prefer a clip of the inferior vena cava. He nearly died after going into shock from bleeding as a complication of his treatment, probably from *anticoagulants*.

Nixon made a full recovery and lived another 19 years, still receiving chronic anti-coagulation therapy. He suffered a stroke and died on April 22, 1994. All five living presidents at the time Jimmy Carter, Gerald Ford, GWH Bush, Ronald Reagan, and Bill Clinton attended his funeral, a presidential first and a show of support for a deceased colleague.

Nixon's medical records are stored in the Nixon Library in Yorba Linda, California. As of June 2021, they were not available to the public.

Gerald Ford 1974-1977 was a football player at the University of Michigan and led a healthy, athletic life, notwithstanding the Chevy Chase caricature on Saturday Night Live that portrayed Ford as an uncoordinated klutz. He was the oldest ex-president at the time of his death at age 93. He survived two separate assassination attempts.

Jimmy Carter 1977-1981: became age 98 on October 1, 2022 and is the oldest living ex-president ever. As of 2023, he is surviving stage IV metastatic melanoma, apparently in remission, supported by state-of-the-art immunotherapy. To date he has avoided the pancreatic cancer that killed his father, brother, and sisters.

Ronald Reagan 1981-1989 survived a serious gunshot wound to the chest at age 70, and was saved by the recently implemented emergency care system at George Washington Hospital.

The transfer of power was sorely tested, since VP Bush was in an airplane. Reagan's staff was confused when Secretary of State Al Haig acclaimed "that as of now I am in charge." In fact, he was in error. Reagan's staff failed to utilize the 25th Amendment but did follow the contingency plans that Reagan had provided beforehand.

Four years later July 1985, Reagan underwent general anesthesia to have surgery for removal of a cancerous colon polyp. He faithfully followed the outline of the 25th Amendment but stated that it did not apply to his situation. The whole process went smoothly, except for Regan's nonsensical statement.

George H.W. Bush 1989-1993: had a major medical illness while president, hyperthyroidism with concurrent atrial fibrillation. This complex medical situation was very well treated by the White House physician, Dr. Burton Lee III. He restored Bush to excellent health with standard medical care.

Bush parachuted from an airplane at ages 80, 85 and 90. He died November 30, 2018, aged 94 years, 5 months, 18 days, and had been the oldest living ex-president at that time. On March 19, 2020, Jimmy Carter overtook him.

Bill Clinton 1993-2001 had significant coronary disease after leaving office. In 2004, he had four vessel coronary bypass surgery. In 2010, he received two coronary stents.

George W. Bush 2001-2009 was healthy. He was the only president to officially activate the 25th Amendment when he twice transferred power to VP Dick Cheney while he underwent colonoscopy.

Barack Obama 2009-2017 was also a healthy man.

Donald Trump 2017-2021 became ill with Covid 19 and was hospitalized for a few days. The details of this illness are not known; only bits of conflicting information were released to the public. He followed in the style of Chester Arthur and JFK, with half-truths and obfuscations. Trump was a major player during the Covid 19 Pandemic of 2020–21. He showed disdain for social distancing, wore a mask in public infrequently, and publicly advocated the injection of bleach as therapy for Covid 19.

Trump had one of his physicians sign a blank piece of professional stationery. Then Trump or his staff composed a letter testifying to his wonderful health and stated that Trump would be the healthiest person ever elected to the presidency. That composition was affixed to the previously signed piece of the doctor's stationery. So much for two hundred years of medical history that stressed the critical importance of accurate medical records.[22]

Finally, Trump refused to accept defeat in the 2020 elections, despite losing over sixty times in court trying to overturn the election results. The US was saved by its independent judiciary.

Joseph Biden 2021-present: The oldest serving president, age 80 November 20, 2022. A survivor of surgery for brain aneurysm in 1987. He has chronic atrial fibrillation for which he receives anti-coagulation therapy. There are apparently no sequelae from any of this.

SERIOUS MEDICAL ILLNESS **has afflicted 19 of the 46 presidents during their time in office.**[23]

- Washington: Abscess thigh, pneumonia
- Madison: Malaria
- Jackson: Lead poisoning, Chronic renal failure
- *Harrison: Probable salmonella enteric infection
- *Taylor: Cholera
- Pierce: Alcoholism, Depression
- Lincoln: Depression
- Arthur: Chronic renal failure
- Cleveland: Oral Cancer
- Wilson: Stroke
- *Harding: Heart Failure, Coronary disease
- Coolidge: Depression
- *F Roosevelt: Hypertension, Heart failure, Angina, Cerebral Hemorrhage
- Eisenhower: Heart attack, Inflammatory bowel disease, Stroke
- Kennedy: Adrenal insufficiency, inflammatory bowel disease
- Johnson: Pneumonia

- Nixon: Thrombophlebitis
- Reagan: Colon Cancer
- George H.W. Bush: Atrial fibrillation, Hyperthyroidism

Four* of those nineteen died in office: W.H. Harrison, Zachary Taylor, Warren Harding, FDR.

8

THE KILLING OF JAMES GARFIELD, OR "IGNORANCE IS BLISS"

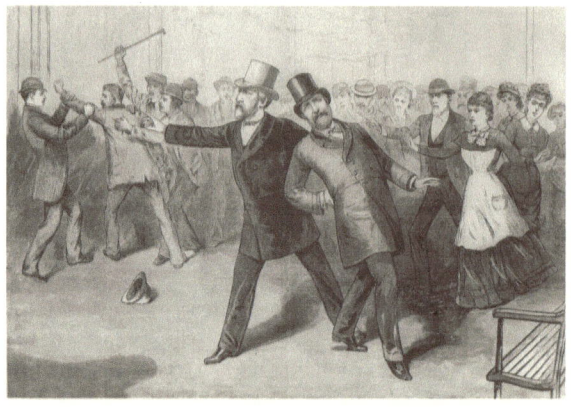

Image 7: Shooting of James Garfield

Despite all of the information coming from Western Europe, despite Semmelweiss and Lister and Koch and Pasteur and John Snow, despite the prevention and control of smallpox, cholera and rabies, the germ theory of disease fell upon deaf ears in the United States in the 1870s to the 1880s. Part of that can be attributed to the poor state of US medical schools, as noted in the Flexner Report of 1910.

Garfield was shot in the right arm and then in his lower

back. His visible twist to the right after being shot in the arm will account for the unusual path of the second bullet in his body.

The medical care received by Garfield was egregious and represents a low point of the history of American medicine. His doctors chose to ignore a mountain of new scientific information that clearly demonstrated that microbes caused infectious disease. They were joined by most of the American medical establishment. The battle of ignorance vs intelligence would be played out over the pus-laden body of James Garfield.

Elected President in 1880, Garfield was a healthy, vigorous 49-year-old man who spent the morning of his assassination jumping around in bed with his young children and doing handstands.[1] Remember this scene seventy-nine days later when Garfield's trip through hell finally ended.

On July 2, 1881, Garfield was about to board a train at the Baltimore and Potomac train station to attend his class reunion at Williams College. He was shot twice by a deranged office seeker who cried out, "Hurrah! Arthur is president!" Chester Arthur was Garfield's vice president but had been his political opponent in the past. The first bullet grazed Garfield's arm, but the other struck his right chest in the lower back and lodged internally. Garfield then fell to the floor.

In the image seen above, Garfield is seen twisting to the right, probably in response to the first gunshot to his right arm.[2] That twist helps explain the unusual path taken by the second bullet, from the right to the left side of his body. By most accounts, he would have lived if left alone with a non-fatal bullet wound.

However, Garfield was killed by his doctors who introduced fatal bacterial infection(s) into his body. At his trial, the assassin claimed, "Your honor, I admit to the shooting of the president, but not the killing." That courtroom plea was probably accurate.

Dr. Townsend was the first to arrive on the scene, and while

Garfield was on the floor of the train station, he probed the back wound with his bare finger and began the process of killing Garfield.[3]

The second physician on the scene was Dr. Charles Purvis, one of only eight black surgeons in the Union Army at the end of the Civil War. At the time of Garfield's shooting, he was surgeon in chief of the Freedman's Hospital in Washington, D.C. Dr. Purvis covered Garfield with some blankets, one of the few instances of anyone providing comfort.

Although several doctors arrived ahead of him, Dr. Doctor W. Bliss took charge, probably because he was accompanied by Robert Todd Lincoln, the former president's son who was then the secretary of war. Robert Todd Lincoln had specifically sought out Dr. Bliss to treat Garfield. He mistakenly gave Bliss credit for being part of the medical team that treated his father's fatal wound. However, Bliss was not involved in Abraham Lincoln's care.[4]

Bliss' parents had named him Doctor Willard Bliss, and after graduation from medical school he was Doctor Doctor Willard Bliss. He had a checkered career and had been a Civil War surgeon, but he was accused of running away from the First Battle of Bull Run. This may be hearsay and is an unproven allegation. He spent most of the Civil War as a hospital administrator, which earned him the praise of Walt Whitman. Bliss was expelled from the District of Columbia Medical Society for opposing the society's exclusion of black physicians. Upon returning to the fold, he embraced the society's opposition to the antiseptic methods that had recently been published by Joseph Lister.

In 1863, he was arrested and briefly imprisoned for accepting a $500 bribe, but the charges were later dropped. He also peddled a concoction called *cudurango* which promised to cure cancer. The medical society accused him of quackery.[5]

Bliss was not the first nor the last doctor to poke his finger into the wound in the president's back, but he was ringmaster for the three-ring circus that soon began. None of the doctors wore surgical gloves, nor did they use clean or sterile instruments.

In *The Destiny of the Republic,* Candice Millard described Bliss's approach and style in treating Garfield. "Bliss selected a long probe that had a white porcelain tip to help locate the bullet. If the tip of the probe came against bone, it would remain white, but a lead bullet would leave a dark mark." X-rays would make these probes obsolete.

These probes could be very painful, but Bliss did not give Garfield anything to ease the pain. Garfield said nothing as Bliss searched for the bullet. "Pressing the unsterilized probe downward and forward into the wound, Bliss did not stop until he had reached a cavity three inches deep in Garfield's back."

Bliss compounded his ignorance with cruelty. At one point the probe became stuck[6] between fractured fragments of the rib, and he was unable to withdraw it. "He finally had to press down on Garfield's fractured rib so that it would lift and release the probe." This caused excruciating pain.

The continued probes of Bliss must be one the most egregious acts of 19th century medicine. The probes never found the bullet, but that did not deter Bliss from continuing to inflict pain upon the president. It became apparent to the most casual observer that these probes were useless and needlessly cruel and caused intense pain. The doctors completed the disgrace with injections of fatal bacteria with every probe.

Dr. Purvis spoke up for the president and for humanity and asked Bliss to end his examination.[8] This was extraordinary bravery for a black man in 1881. Bliss continued to probe, and Purvis was unable to stop him. Bliss's outrageous behavior was contrary to the teachings of the past several centuries. Medical care needs to be humane, focusing upon the comfort of the patient. The pain must have been terrific, but Garfield received no morphine until the second day. After Garfield's repeated insistence, he was finally moved to the White House.

During his seventy-nine days of agony, probes were repeated by Dr. Bliss and by about fourteen other doctors. The president had received a non-fatal bullet wound, but was done in by each of the doctors who repeatedly stuck their dirty fingers into his back wound, introducing a fatal bacterial infection with each and every digital probe. They continued to do so throughout the course of his illness. These repeated probes were obscene.

About twenty doctors examined Garfield, first at the train station and later at the White House. Fifteen of them would probe the back wound with their finger. How did they justify putting their dirty finger into the president's wound while he was lying on the filthy floor of a train station? Perhaps these doctors had not heard of the germ theory or had never heard of Lister.

The basic problem was that Garfield's doctors knew about the germ theory of infectious disease but did not accept it despite overwhelming evidence supporting it.

There is a striking similarity between modern day deniers of climate change and of US physicians who were opposed to the germ theory of infection. The anti-science movement in the US, is now 300 years old and going strong.

None of the groups in 1721, 1881 or today trust science and the scientific method. They disregard the large body of scientific evidence placed before them by a group of eminent international scientists. Despite all the scientific progress, Dr. Bliss and friends seemed oblivious to the germ theory and to Jenner, Holmes, Semmelweis, Snow, Lister, Koch, and Pasteur. They just could not believe that doctors were the vectors of surgical infection.

In *The Murder of James A. Garfield*, James C. Clark says, "Surgical conditions were often filthy, and doctors took some pride in the filth." [9] It was said that "every surgeon was proud of his old operating coat, which he neither washed nor changed. Doctors wore the same coat from surgery to surgery, proudly displaying their blood encrusted wares. The accumulated incrustation of dried blood and pus attested to the doctor's experience, like accumulated service stripes on a soldier's uniform." That sentiment exemplified the opposition to the germ theory of disease

In retrospect, this is not surprising considering the poor state of US medical schools. The Flexner report of 1910 gave them a failing grade overall. Too many of them were proprietary schools with minimal clinical education at the bedside. Few had any academic affiliation, and the curriculum was not steeped in the modern science of the 19th century. Only Johns Hopkins was on a par with the great European universities and only a few other American schools were close. No wonder American doctors were slow to accept the germ theory.

During the Garfield malpractice melodrama, one cringes to learn that Garfield remained fully conscious throughout the multiple probings. There had been no attempt to protect his privacy, and only minimal effort to provide some comfort. Finally, in an act of kindness, someone placed him on a horsehair mattress instead of being left directly on the floor of a train station right in front of the women's restrooms.

But doctors continued to pass by and probe his wound with their dirty fingers without hardly any introduction. This recalls the preposterous scene from Monty Python: *"We are here for your liver."* How could the president of the US be so humiliated?

Under the influence of Florence Nightingale and Joseph Lister, the modern hospital was rapidly evolving into a place of cleanliness, comfort, and healing. Garfield was never taken to hospital but was eventually taken to the White House where he at least gained some privacy. George Washington University Hospital had been open since 1824, and that locale would have been a marked improvement over the floor of the train station or even the White House which was not much better with its "leaking pipes and rotten beams."[10]

Since the Battle of Gettysburg in 1863, the standard of care for wounded men was rapid evacuation to hospital by ambulance. Medical triage and rapid transport to hospital was the standard of care for treating bullet wounds in 1881. Shouldn't the president get care equal to or better than an army private?

The doctors persisted, with their unclean fingers and instruments, to torture Garfield with more useless and fatal probes and drains. None of these probes took place in a hospital operating room. The wound soon became a super-infected, pus-ridden, gash of human flesh, beginning at the right posterior ribs and extending to the right groin.

Navy Surgeon General Wales stuck his finger in the wound and proclaimed the bullet had hit the president's liver. Not only was he incorrect, but his exam and that of others led to an eventual abscess in the area around the liver. During his seventy-nine days of agony, Garfield was continually examined with unwashed fingers and unsterile probes.

Garfield was shot in 1881, five years after Lister's US tour and several years after Koch and Pasteur proved that bacteria caused disease.[11] There was no excuse for the ignorance of Dr. Bliss and company. This was beyond ordinary malpractice and was another low point in the history of American medicine.[12]

Some days after the shooting, Garfield's personal doctor, White House physician Dr. Jedediah Baxter, arrived on the scene. Dr. Baxter and Dr. Bliss promptly had a shoving match and fought over the patient, the president of the United States who lay in bed in agony. Baxter backed down, left Bliss in charge, and never saw the president again.

Despite all this medical malpractice, Garfield's assassination is associated with three scientific inventions, brought about to expedite Garfield's care and to alleviate his suffering.[13]

. . .

Invention #1: The air conditioner

As the summer heat continued, Garfield was suffering from a scorching fever, relentless chills, and increasing confusion. The summer of 1881 was also unusually hot in Washington. Schemes immediately developed to keep the president cool and comfortable during his recovery. The explorer John Wesley Powell and the polymath Simon Newcomb invented and built an air conditioner specifically to provide relief for Garfield. It was the first ever air conditioner and functioned fairly well, lowering the room temperature by 20 degrees F.

Here is another perspective of how far behind the curve were Garfield's doctors. In 1881, the same year that Bliss stuck his dirty fingers into Garfield, Newcomb was working on experiments to measure the speed of light. It was as though Bliss and Newcomb were from different planets, although they lived at the same time, in the same city.

Having exhausted the limits of their own fingers, the physicians were ready to pass their search for the bullet into the hands of technology.

Invention #2: The metal detector

Alexander Graham Bell invented the metal detector specifically to find the bullet in President Garfield.[14] He brought it to the White House on July 26, some three weeks after the shooting.

Bell's device had two electromagnets connected to a telephone receiver that would click when a metal object passed between the magnets. In any event, it didn't find the bullet because the metal springs in Garfield's bed distorted the results. Also, Dr. Bliss allowed Bell to only use the device on Garfield's right side. The doctors had made the false assumption that a bullet that entered the right side of the back had to be on the right side of the abdomen.[15]

Bell's subsequent tests indicated that his metal detector was in good working order. In fact, his metal detector would be the prototype for the land mine detectors used in World War I. The attempt of Bell to find the bullet with his newly invented metal detector has to be seen as cutting-edge science of the 19th century.

INVENTION #3: **The water bed**

Fed up with the heat, Garfield dictated that he be moved to the New Jersey shore in the vain hope that the fresh air and quiet there might aid his recovery. On September 6, Garfield was transported while lying on a waterbed that was specifically invented and built to lessen the bumps of the journey. The fates were conspiring against Garfield, since the Jersey shore was suffering the greatest heat wave in twenty years. The move did little to improve his condition.

Garfield's diet was not for a man with a poor stomach. Every day he received beefsteak, eggs, and brandy.[16] He was vomiting continuously, losing 80 pounds in six short weeks. So, his doctors opted for a nutritional enema.[17]

They mixed together an egg, one ounce of bouillon, one and a half ounces of milk, a half ounce of whiskey, and ten drops of opium and inserted this concoction into the president's rectum. Needless to say, this strategy proved ineffective. Rectal absorption of undigested food has not been shown to occur in humans. That did not stop Dr. Bliss from writing a book promoting rectal feeding.

Garfield's doctors released promising news to the press but recorded their dismal outlook in private journals. Was this the beginning of a cover-up? The press, to its credit, quickly grew skeptical of the reports and suspected the president's death was near. They were close to the truth as the infection raged within Garfield's system.

Voluminous amounts of pus drained from Garfield's chest wound, and his face grew large and puffy as a salivary gland filled with more pus. By August 19, his right eye had swollen shut. On August 30, several incisions were made in his face to facilitate drainage. Pus ran from most of his orifices and he nearly drowned in his own secretions. As the doctors argued over the bullet's location and what to do about it, Garfield lingered for 79 days, conducting state business from his bed. Was Garfield really able to discharge the "Powers and Duties of the said Office?" By now he was delirious much of the time.

News of Garfield's shooting flew around the country. Telegrams poured into the White House offering ideas. One suggested hanging the president upside down and allowing the bullet to fall out. Another urged that a rubber tube be inserted into the wound, attached to an air pump, and the bullet removed by suction. Many newspapers had front-page cartoons displaying the president's agony in detail. The newspaper coverage was continuous, graphic, sensational, and lurid.

The Garfields had no privacy from the press. Should the president have had any expectations of privacy? Didn't the press have an obligation to find out the truth about the president's health, regardless of the invasion of privacy? Was it fair for the press to detail all the intimate details of Garfield's tribulations to the waiting world?

Two days before he died, Garfield summarized his feelings about everything that transpired. He wrote the following on a calling card, *"Strangulates pro republica,"* which translates to "tortured for the Republic."[18]

Garfield deteriorated further and after 79 days of agony, died on September 19, 1881.

The family agreed to an autopsy and that is where the doctors found that they had blundered. The bullet was not on the right side of Garfield's abdomen, it was on the left.[19]

IN THE IMAGE BELOW, follow the dotted line on top to see the path of the bullet. The bullet entered the right lower chest and shattered the eleventh right rib. Its path was now deflected toward the left. At the midline it passed through the body of the first lumbar vertebra, missing the spinal cord and the great veins and arteries of the lower abdomen. The bullet continued on a leftward trajectory, coming to rest in a collection of fat, located posterior to the pancreas.

The bullet did not injure the pancreas, and apparently the bullet also missed the spleen. This was a magic bullet delivering a non-lethal gunshot wound, laying quietly behind the pancreas, minding its own business and doing no harm. There was also a great deal of infection around the gallbladder. An abscess, probably caused by the doctors, was found in the vicinity of the gallbladder, between the liver and the transverse colon. The doctors had been searching for the bullet on the right side of Garfield, when in fact, it was on his left side behind the pancreas. All their probes had been in vain, worse than useless, since they had injected lethal doses of bacteria into Garfield.

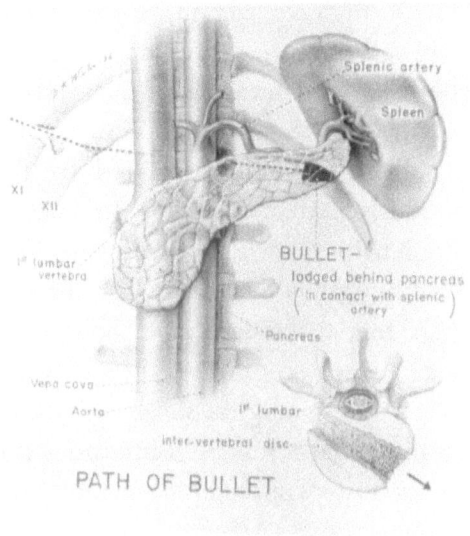

Image 8: RIGHT - LEFT - Garfield's autopsy; Body on its back, facing the reader.

A LONG PUS-FILLED channel extended from the external wound on his lower right back, between the loin muscles and the right kidney, almost to the right groin. This channel was not the track of the bullet, but instead was created by the doctors' probings. The doctors had turned a three-inch-deep, harmless entrance wound into a twenty-inch-long contaminated canal. This was the source of the *sepsis* that killed him.

The autopsy also found an injury to the *splenic* artery and some blood in the abdominal cavity. Was this the immediate cause of death and, if so, when did it occur? How did it occur? Was it related in some way to the overwhelming infections?

DESPITE THE OCCURRENCE of medical malpractice, modern science came onto the scene with the first working air conditioner, the first metal detector, and the first water mattress. All were invented and employed to enhance Garfield's care. How do you explain Dr. Bliss and Simon Newcomb, the first representing ignorance, the second representing the cutting edge of science, and both involved in caring for Garfield?

Vice President Chester Arthur was horrified by the lack of privacy and public humiliation suffered by the Garfields. Arthur was seriously ill during his time in office, but he organized a comprehensive cover-up that kept his illness a secret. He did not want his family to suffer as had the Garfields. This became the presidential standard until the time of Eisenhower's heart attack.

Garfield's death from surgical sepsis was the Waterloo for the opponents of the germ theory of infectious disease. There was no going back. Lister's opponents were finished.

Another question comes to mind. It was well known by 1881 that there were hundreds if not thousands of Civil War combat veterans surviving and doing well with bullets embedded in a wide variety of bodily locations.[20] So why perform all this probing to remove the bullet?

The assassin attempted to defend himself in court, but was convicted and hanged.

9
TALE OF TWO PAINTINGS

Two paintings by the American master Thomas Eakins (1844-1918) can be appreciated on several levels, the artistic and the historical. Let's accept that they are great pieces of art and focus upon the historical content. Although he does not appear on either canvas, these works as a group could be called the Triumph of Joseph Lister.

The Gross Clinic by Thomas Eakins is a masterpiece of 19th century American art. Dr. Gross was a renowned teacher and surgeon at the Jefferson Medical College in Philadelphia, and president of the American Medical Association.

Dr. Gross pauses during the surgery and appears to be making a teaching point, which is probably a demonstration of his new technique for treating osteomyelitis, a sign of modernity. Instead of amputating the young man's leg, he does only local surgery in order to treat the apparent bone infection. He appears ready to point his bloody hand to emphasize a point that he is making. In this one instant of time, one of surgery's major teaching techniques can be seen:

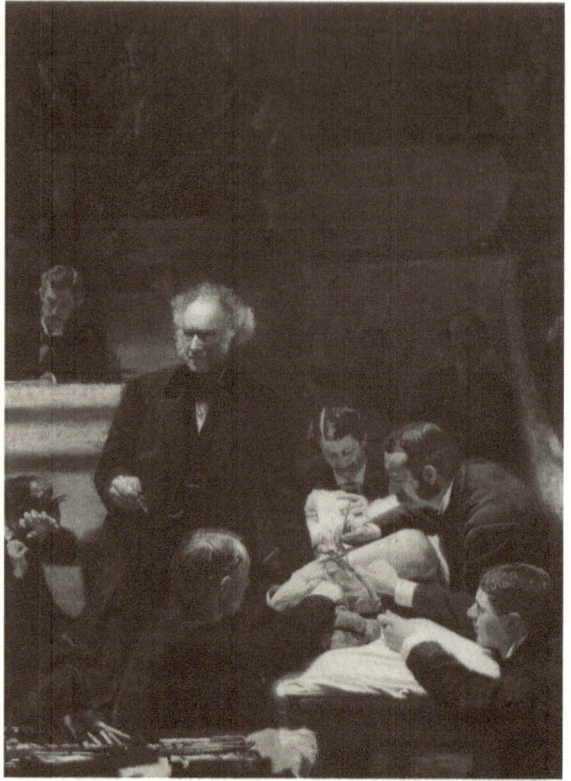

Image 9: The Gross Clinic, *by Thomas Eakins, 1875, The Philadelphia Museum of Art;*

For the students in the background "See one"
For Dr. Gross "Do one"
For Dr. Gross "Teach one"

ANOTHER POINT of modernity is that the patient is receiving ether anesthesia. There is also a clerk recording the operative notes. This is following the Pierre Louis school that emphasized medical measurements and recording that information.

However, this painting does not look like a modern operating room. It is from the end of the late 1800s. Great change is about to occur, but you would never know it by looking at this painting, which appears to be locked in time from a long while back. It is too dark; no light source is visible. All the visible light is from sunlight coming through unseen skylights. There were no electric lights as they would not be commercially available in the US until after November 1879, when Thomas Edison received his US patent, four years after Dr. Gross was painted. The surgeons are all wearing street clothes rather than surgical gowns and gloves.

The medical instruments are displayed on the table and not in any sort of sterile container. A woman is sitting off to the side of the surgeons, probably a relative of the patient who is there to safeguard the patient, whether dead or alive. Is she coughing and spraying her germs all over the room or is she just turning away her gaze? If the patient died during surgery, she wanted to be sure that the body would be taken for a proper burial and not be secreted off by grave robbers, who sold bodies to the medical schools for anatomy lessons.

Samuel Gross heard Lister lecture in 1876 in Philadelphia. At the time he was a man of great prestige, professor of surgery at Jefferson Medical College and president of the American Medical Association. His support of Lister would have had great impact; however, he was unimpressed. He was quoted as saying, "Little if any faith is placed by any enlightened or experienced surgeon on this side of the Atlantic in the so-called carbolic acid treatment of Professor Lister."[1]

Samuel Gross did not operate on Garfield, but his failure to support Lister gave a cover of respect and authority to Dr. Bliss and company. Garfield's surgeons probably felt they were following the standard of care, supported by physicians of the stature of Samuel Gross.

President Garfield suffered for 79 days and died because the US medical leadership opposed the germ theory. After Garfield's death, the country and the world was aghast when the surgeon's blunders were exposed at autopsy.

The Dr. Gross painting represents surgery before the era of

Lister. There was total disregard for the germ theory of infectious disease. In fact, the painting glorifies Dr. Gross with his heroic pose and the light focused upon his forehead.

Eakins entered the Dr. Gross painting to be exhibited at the 1876 Philadelphia Centennial Exposition. It was turned down. Eakins apparently received no monetary composition for this work. In 2006, the citizens of Philadelphia and Wells Fargo Bank paid $68 million for the painting to remain in Philadelphia.

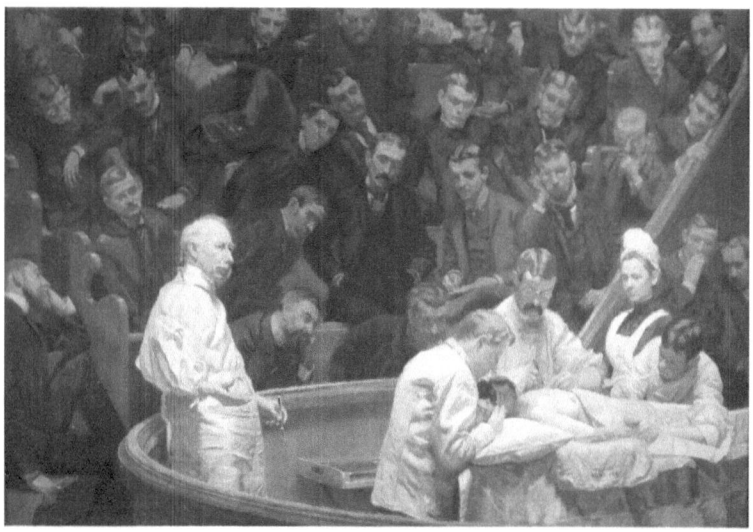

Image 10: The Agnew Clinic, Thomas Eakins, U of Pennsylvania Medical School, Philadelphia, 1889

The Agnew Clinic the second painting in our tale. Note how much brighter this picture is. Surgical illumination is now by electric lights, commercially available since 1879. The patient's relative is no longer present, and there will be no more danger from her spewing germs into the operating room, while coughing or crying or sneezing.

There are hospital drapes for the operation. All the operating room (OR) staff are in surgical white gowns, except for the nurse, Mary Clymer, who is wearing a white apron. The presence of an OR nurse is testament to the rising professional status of nurses. Besides Agnew, she is the only person standing erect. Her presence in the operating room is a sign of modernity.

Surgical instruments are seen only in the hands of the surgeons. The remainder are probably in the metal case that's seen near Dr. Agnew's left hand. The anesthesia is being administered via a cone, a modern improvement. The patient's breast is exposed, as the operation is a partial *mastectomy*. Eakins was very interested in painting the human body.

But most incredible is the presence of Dr. Agnew, who occupies a place of prominence as though he had been the champion of the aseptic technique of surgery. History says otherwise. This painting serves several purposes.

The Dr. Agnew painting of 1889 demonstrated the integrity of the intact hospital surgical unit, experienced surgeon in full surgical gear, sterile operating room, available equipment on site, a trained team, all leading to a good outcome for operations. Presidents McKinley and Cleveland will be denied that opportunity for dubious reasons.

This was Dr. Agnew's last hurrah at the University of Pennsylvania. The painting was a tribute to his career as a teacher. Like Dr. Gross, he is standing away from the operating table as though ready to make some teaching points for his audience, the medical school graduating class of 1889, seen in the background. This is their class portrait. Eakins was well paid for this painting, a $750 commission paid by the students at the medical school. The theme of each painting is the same: "a teaching moment in surgery." Yet, the surgical world had turned upside down in the interval.

The Gross Clinic reflected the days before the acceptance of germ theory, *The Agnew Clinic* reflected the acceptance and glory of aseptic surgery. Dr. Gross appears to be from ancient times. *The Agnew Clinic* looks like a modern operating room.

And yet these painting are only fourteen years apart. Change comes about slowly, very slowly and then—bang! All at once.

The Dr. Gross painting focuses upon the surgeon, who is the largest and most central figure of the painting. In the Dr. Agnew painting, the surgeon is off to the side. He is not larger than anyone else and the focus is on the operating table. The scene is lit up by electric lights that had been installed. The brightness of the painting asks us to view this scene as the "enlightenment" received from Lister and Pasteur. Can Dr. Gross and Dr. Bliss be thought of as creatures who are in the dark? This is how this modern-day physician views these paintings.

Dr. David Agnew of the University of Pennsylvania Medical School was one of President Garfield's doctors. He was called into consultation on July 3, 1881. From that time forward, he was the chief surgical consultant for Dr. Bliss and faithfully remained in attendance at the patient's bedside for much of the 79 days.

He must share blame for the many blunders committed by the surgical team. Good intentions and diligence were not enough. By failing to adopt antisepsis, the doctors were injecting fatal doses of bacteria into Garfield. All their good intentions were overcome by this fatal flaw in their management. Like Benjamin Rush one hundred years before, they worked very hard at doing the wrong thing.

There is no evidence that Agnew did any probing of the bullet wound, but there was no evidence that he stopped any of the probes. He did, however, perform surgery.[2] Garfield's case became increasingly complicated as collections of pus began appearing that required drainage. The team of doctors went so far as to put Garfield under ether anesthesia and explore the right side of his abdomen. They drained an abscess and placed two drains in his abdomen that were blindly advanced into his body. This surgery with unwashed instruments and unwashed hands and blind probes was performed by Dr. Agnew, who apparently did not yet subscribe to the theory of antisepsis in 1881.[3]

A photograph of Dr. Agnew in surgery taken in 1888 showed him dressed in a buttoned-up street coat, but it also appears that carbolic acid was being used during surgery. Dr. Agnew was beginning to embrace antiseptic surgery. Consider him partially converted to Lister in 1888.

In 1889, he is in full aseptic mode. He has fully embraced the aseptic technique for his portrait, where he is wearing a surgical gown and where carbolic acid does not appear. When Dr. Agnew was painted in 1889, his conversion was complete. Lister's theories had prevailed, and that can be seen in the aseptic set up of the surgeons and operating room.

Those who opposed Lister were swept away by the advances in Europe of Pasteur and Koch. Somehow Dr. Agnew's reputation survived, and he thrived. He defended Dr. Bliss and the physicians' care of Garfield, and yet he avoided significant criticism. Instead, he would be glorified by Eakins for eternity, standing there in full aseptic surgical gown. Thomas Eakins gave cover to David Agnew, hiding him in plain sight. Art history appears to enshrine Agnew as a champion of scientific progress, when the truth yields a mixed result.

Both these paintings are wonderful illustrations of medical history. The hero of the story is Joseph Lister, but he doesn't get an Eakins portrait. Perhaps Eakins' choice of Agnew was meant to be ironic. But then again, Eakins was well paid to do the Dr. Agnew painting.

But someone else is missing from the paintings. That someone is President James Garfield. Unless you are an art historian, he is the reason we are interested in these back stories. By suffering through his trial by infection, he gave up his life, and that led to the final triumph for germ theory. That triumph was enshrined forever by *The Agnew Clinic*.

When Garfield's autopsy was made public, it yielded the

information that led to the final triumph of Lister and the germ theory. Garfield had not died in vain.

MANY THREADS INTERSECTED in the murder of Garfield: Garfield's assassination at the hands of a rejected office seeker led to the reform of the civil service; the transfer of power by murder led to the new Succession Act of 1886; the failure to provide relief for a disabled president led eventually to the 25th Amendment; the asynchrony between Dr Bliss and Joseph Lister exemplified the inherent conflicts seen throughout our timetable; the failure to appreciate the benefits of hospitalization continued for Presidents McKinley, Wilson, Harding, Cleveland, and Nixon.

President Garfield was cared for by the morally-marginal Dr. Doctor Bliss, the distinguished Dr. David Agnew, the inventor Alexander Graham Bell, the explorer John Wesley Powell, the polymath Simon Newcomb, and the black surgeon Dr. Charles Purvis. This eclectic group of care-givers embodies the overarching themes of scientific discovery, exploration and expansion of the American West, racial justice and prejudice, and post-bellum partisan politics that have moved our story along its time line. A nice touch was that Garfield the abolitionist was treated by Purvis, a free black man born to free black parents.

10

LESS THAN BEST MEDICAL CARE

The failure to provide excellent medical care for every president is a mystery. In several instances it was the failure of someone to yell, "STOP! This is not right." But too often a strong personality triumphed over wiser minds.

Eight presidents received less than best medical care. Eisenhower's substandard care only lasted twelve hours; afterwards, he received excellent care. FDR's substandard care was the failure of his physician to make the initial diagnosis of heart failure. That was followed by excellent care by his cardiologist, Dr. Howard Bruenn. Kennedy's substandard care was intertwined with a lot of very good care, which would prevail. JFK, Eisenhower, and FDR will each be discussed in a separate chapter. The incredible malpractice foisted upon James Garfield has already been discussed in chapter 8.

But there remain five presidents who require further discussion.

1. The death of George Washington, whose doctors followed the 1799 standard of heroic medical care.

2. The lunacy of performing dangerous surgery on Grover Cleveland while cruising up the East River in New York Harbor.

3. The failure of expediency to provide adequate care for William McKinley.

4. The folly of sending a very sick Warren Harding to a hotel room instead of to hospital.

5. We will also include the coverup by Chester Arthur of his chronic kidney disease, whose medical care otherwise seemed adequate.

The Death of Washington.

Washington's final illness demonstrated the failure of the entire heroic medical system, which lagged behind the cutting edge of 18th century science.

To have a meaningful discussion about medical competence, we need to remember the standard of care during the time in question.

George Washington's doctors cannot be held to modern standards of care. We can help orient ourselves by placing the events in the proper context of time. Instead of making a judgment about the quality of care in 1799, the events of the day will be laid out for your consideration.

Friday morning, December 13, 1799, former President George Washington (GW) awoke with a sore throat. He became hoarse and retired early. He awakened the next day, December 14 at 2 a.m. with a sore neck, fever and chills, and could hardly speak. He was breathing with great difficulty and would be dead before the day was done.[1]

Against the wishes of Martha, the decision was made to proceed with bloodletting and approximately fourteen ounces were removed. Long-time friend and former Surgeon General of the Army, Dr. James Craik, arrived at 9 a.m. and induced a second bleeding of a quart of blood, and repeated the same at 11 a.m. With no noticeable improvement, *blistering* was induced by a flannel dipped in *cantharides* (a preparation of crushed beetles), wrapped around the neck. A gargle concoction of vinegar and sage tea was administered to provide some relief for the sore throat. At noon an *enema* was given. This was *"heroic medicine"* at its worst multiple bloodlettings, blistering, and enemas.

Martha Washington became more alarmed and requested a second opinion. Dr. Gustavos Brown arrived at 3 p.m., the same time as did another young physician, Dr. Elisha Dick. Drs. Craik and Brown favored a fourth bleeding which was performed over the objections of Dr. Dick. By then Washington's doctors removed 80 ounces of blood or thirty-five percent of his blood volume, an extraordinary amount even by 1799 standards. Note that two of the participants on the scene were opposed to bloodletting, Dr. Dick and Martha Washington.

Dr. Dick made the plea that Washington should not be depleted of any more of his blood but should undergo tracheotomy for what he thought was an inflammation of the throat membranes. Since 1718, tracheotomy had been accepted in Europe as a means to relieve obstructed airways, although it was infrequently performed. Dr. Dick may have seen the procedure and was ready to do this one.

This complied with the action-oriented theory of medical education regarding procedures: *"See one. Do one. Teach one."* This was still the unwritten code at Boston City Hospital in 1969, where I did some training. Supporting this theory of education are the following corollaries:

Pay attention in class, by the bedside, and during procedures. Sick patients require a sense of urgency and not a long philosophic debate. Physicians are obliged to pass on knowledge to the next generation of physicians.

Dr. Dick's plea for tracheotomy was overruled by Dr. Craik, the senior physician of the group, a man of great prestige, and a long-time friend of GW. Undoubtedly, the specter of failure of the procedure upon the most famous person in America, if not the world, weighed heavily in the decision to veto the procedure. GW died at approximately 10:22 p.m. while taking his own pulse.

The following morning, another local physician, Dr. William Thornton, sent a message asking for permission to do a postmortem tracheotomy to try to resuscitate GW, but that offer was turned down.

Twenty years after Washington's death, Dr. Thornton wrote that when the former president was suffering through his final illness, a family member invited him to Mount Vernon to see if he could help. He was shocked to discover that Washington had died before his arrival. But Thornton had a backup plan. "The weather was very cold & he (Washington) remained in a frozen state for several Days. I proposed to attempt his restoration in the following manner: First to thaw him in cold water, then lay him in blankets, and then by degrees and by friction to give him warmth, and to put into activity the minute blood vessels, and at the same time open a passage to the Lungs by the Trachea, and to inflate them with air, to produce an artificial respiration, and to transfuse blood into him (from a lamb). Washington died by the loss of blood & the want of air. (...) and there was no doubt in my mind that his restoration was possible."[2]

Resuscitation of a dead and frozen person is not a farfetched idea. The doctors in 18th century Virginia had heard of occasional accounts of young men, usually slaves, who were found partially submerged in freezing creeks and presumed to be dead from drowning. They would be taken to the main house to prepare for burial. On rare occasions, while rewarming indoors, these slaves would awaken to the astonishment of all.

In the 21st century, no one who is severely hypothermic is ever pronounced dead, no matter how dead they may appear. Severe hypothermia slows down the vital signs so much that a patient may appear lifeless. The benefits of rewarming are well known in the 21st century. Not until the hypothermic patient is warmed up and/or has an EKG will doctors state whether the patient is dead. That did not pertain for Washington, because he had been warming up in-doors for a few days and was no longer hypothermic when he was pronounced dead.

Some conclusions can be drawn. In northern Virginia, in December 1799, there were at least two physicians, Dr. Dick and Dr. Thornton, prepared to do a tracheotomy. Dr. Thornton correctly stated that Washington died because he was very cold, he had lost blood from four bloodlettings, and he could not get air into his lungs to breathe. Dr. Thornton basically prescribed CPR and tracheotomy. Pretty good for 1799.

This was not surprising, since Thornton was a graduate of the University of Edinburgh, probably the best medical school in the world at the time. Dr. Craik also studied at the University of Edinburgh, and had been physician general of the Continental Army. Dr. Dick graduated from the University of Pennsylvania. So, Washington's doctors were among the best educated in the world.

All of Washington's doctors correctly agreed that he had an inflammatory process in the throat. By today's medical assessment,[3] Washington showed the classic features of acute *epiglottitis*, a rapidly progressive infectious disease, characterized by severe pain and difficulty breathing, talking, and swallowing.

The following represents modern thinking about the death of Washington, as proposed by Dr. White M. Wallenborn. "The epiglottis is located at the base of the tongue and at the entrance to the airway. When infected it swells up and blocks the airway, causing death. Diphtheria is also possible diagnosis, but less likely since GW probably had diphtheria as a child. Tracheotomy would have been the appropriate therapy for either diphtheria or epiglottis, since antibiotics were not available in 1799."[3]

It is difficult for a 21st century doctor to pass meaningful judgment on any of Washington's physicians. His doctors had made a good diagnosis, at least close enough. One of the ongoing issues in medicine is that the standard of care often lags behind the cutting edge of science, as true today as it was in 1799. Not doing a tracheotomy was the standard of care in 1799. Doing a tracheotomy was on the cutting edge in 1799.

In the *Philadelphia Medical and Physical Journal* published in 1809, Dr. Dick commented that he was not in agreement with the treatment plans that ...day in 1799. " Re: the death of Washington ... death was inevitable unless it could be arrested by the operation of tracheotomy, ... as the only expedient that could possibly preserve the life of the man ... I shall never cease to regret that the operation was not performed."[4]

Why did Dr. Craik, who was in-charge, fail to implement the new technology? We can only speculate because he did not record his reasons. It may be very difficult to make critical medical decisions for lifelong friends, especially to perform radical surgery.

It is another good reason not to choose a physician because he is a good friend. This is the first time, but not the last, that treating one's friends becomes an issue. In Washington's case, there may have been another reason that a tracheotomy was not done. Dr Craik may not have had the nerve due to the immense fame of George Washington, despite the fact that Washington was clearly dying. Why not try a *tracheotomy?* Perhaps Dr. Craik did not want to be known as the doctor who killed Washington, which ironically was to be his fate. That judgment is incorrect and not justified.

WILLIAM MCKINLEY IS **unplugged (electrically)**

President William McKinley had taken the US onto the world stage and stood at the height of his political power. After War with Spain in 1898, the US acquired and occupied its new empire in the Pacific. In 1900, McKinley was re-elected president and Teddy Roosevelt became his VP.

But in 1901, he received surgical care that was not state of the art and could have been better; instead, it was less than best. It demonstrated the difference between what was expedient and what could or should have been outstanding care.

On September 6, 1901, President McKinley was in Buffalo, New York, attending the Pan American Exposition that featured many recent scientific and electrical discoveries. Buffalo was an appropriate site, as electrical power had been generated from the nearby waters of Niagara Falls since 1882. After the opening of the power plant at the Falls in 1895, it became possible to bring electricity 22 miles to Buffalo by the use of alternating current (AC) and high voltage transmission lines. This was the work of Nikola Tesla.[5]

Buffalo and other distant sites were now able to receive electricity from the Falls and use it for multiple tasks, including lighting lamps, moving streetcars, and numerous other operations. The use of AC electricity at the Pan-American Exposition in 1901 was fundamental to the success of the fair.

From the October 1901 issue of *Everybody's Magazine,* "Other newly developed technologies on display were the portable X-ray machine, the electrograph, which was a device that transmitted pictures over a wire, a voting machine, a typesetting machine, an improved phonograph; and infant incubators, with real infants inside." There were also electric ambulances on site.[6]

The Pan-American Exposition was an extravaganza worthy of the name of world's fair, and the wonders of electricity were the highlight. All the buildings were electrified and lit up at night, the highlight being the Electric Tower. Unfortunately, it was on the grounds of this exposition that the president of the United States would be assassinated.

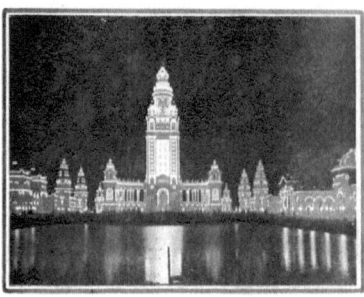

Image 11: The Pan American Exposition, Buffalo, New York, 1901 was completely electrified. The highlight was the The Electric Tower

On September 6, 1901 at 4:07 p.m. McKinley was greeting the public on a receiving line. The assassin made his way to the front of the line, slapped away the president's outstretched hand, pointed a gun at the president's midsection, and fired twice.

One bullet deflected off McKinley's rib cage and did no damage. The other bullet went through the president's stomach, kidney, and pancreas before settling in his back. It took nearly forty minutes for the first physician, Herman Mynter to arrive on the scene. He was a general surgeon from Buffalo and began his surgical evaluation of McKinley at the Exposition's first aid station.

After Mynter's initial examination was finished, Dr. Matthew Mann arrived on the scene. He was a former dean of Buffalo Medical School and a respected gynecologist and obstetrician. This former dean had a lot of prestige, but he was not a general surgeon.

After Mynter and Mann conferred, it was agreed that Dr. Mann would perform a surgical exploration of McKinley at the exposition *first aid station*. They did not go to the well-equipped Buffalo General Hospital via the on-site electric ambulances a quick 15-minute trip. Instead, after obtaining McKinley's consent, they elected to do the surgery at the first aid station. This became a critical error.

The first aid station had two major deficiencies. There were no surgical retractors to be found on site. Retractors are surgical instruments that widen and enlarge the area beneath the surgical incision to allow visualization of the organs within.

Also, the first aid station was not wired for electricity, so there were no electric lights. The irony of the situation is that the Pan American exposition was mainly about the wonders of electricity. There were electrical exhibits and electricity everywhere except in the room used to do surgery on the president of the United States. Expediency had been mistaken for efficiency.

It was already late afternoon and almost dusk when the surgery began. The surgical field was illuminated by the fading late afternoon sunlight, reflected onto the operative field from mirrors and metal basins, held up by medical staff. After an hour of surgery, a working electric light finally made its way to the aid station.

Visualization of the operative field was impaired by several factors. The lighting was very dim. Retractors were not available to widen the operation site. Mc Kinley's obese abdomen added another degree of difficulty for visualization of the operative site. The surgeons had to go through three inches of fat to reach the abdominal cavity. How could Dr. Mann see what he was doing? He was later quoted as saying, "that it was like operating at the darkened end of a big hole." Doing surgery on an obese man without retractors in the fading late afternoon sun is less than best medical care.

Instead of waiting 40 minutes for a physician to appear, the president should have been taken immediately via an on-site electric ambulance to Buffalo General Hospital. The trip to the hospital by electric ambulance would have taken about 15 to 20 minutes, less than the 40 minutes spent waiting for Dr. Mynter to arrive at the first aid station. The standard of care since the Battle of Gettysburg was for rapid evacuation to a hospital. There had been electricity in Buffalo since 1895, so it is safe to surmise that the Buffalo General Hospital had electric lights. At the hospital, electric lighting, retractors and full surgical kit, trained surgical teams, and the presence of aseptic surgery were available.

Ironically, one of the best general surgeons in the US, Dr. Roswell Park, was on the staff of Buffalo General Hospital. However, at that moment he was in the middle of *neck dissection* surgery at Niagara Falls Memorial Hospital about fourteen miles away. Almost as soon as the president had been shot, a telegraph messenger was sent to him. As described years later by Dr. Park's son, the messenger ran into the operating room and told Dr. Park that he was needed immediately.

Park responded, "Don't you see I am in the middle of a case. I can't leave even if it were for the president of the United States." The messenger replied, "Doctor, it is for the president of the United States." But Park proceeded to finish the operation before going to the president. For Dr. Park, his patient on the operating room table had priority over the president.

But because the president was the patient, a special express train was sent to Niagara Falls to pick up Dr. Park when he finished his surgery and take him to Buffalo. Park finally arrived at the first aid station as Mann was sewing up the incision. Mann had cleaned the wound and searched in vain for the bullet. He asked Park if any drains need be placed in the abdomen. Dr. Park left that decision for Dr. Mann, who decided not to drain the abdomen since there appeared to be no excess blood or fluid. It was the expediency of doing surgery at the exposition first aid station that was the major deficiency.[7]

During the surgery, an aide to the president sent out a request to have the X-ray machine at the fair brought to McKinley. The machine was not sent, however, since the surgical team felt that using the machine might cause undue stress on the president and that the X-ray might not prove of much value even if taken. Since 1900, X-ray machines had been in general use in clinical practice and did not cause stress for patients. They also worked very well for locating bullets.

This major failure to implement modern care occurred at the same time the US was in the middle of rapidly expanding technological progress. The electrical revolution was in full bloom. The world was beginning to reap the benefits of the germ theory. Nevertheless, the president of the US was subjected to sub-standard surgical care.

How can a doctor agree to operate in a room without electric lights? How can he do abdominal surgery on an obese man without retractors? It was as though the revolution in hospital care had not taken place.

Park and his surgical team at Buffalo General was the correct way to go. Everything was in place except for a designated decision maker. Instead of taking the president to the first aid station, the need was for someone to yell out, "Get the president to Buffalo General by the electric ambulance." The failure to do just that cost McKinley his life.

In 1981, US Secret Service Special Agent Jerry Parr, under similar circumstances when President Reagan was shot, would issue the appropriate command. "Go to George Washington Hospital." That was the crucial decision that saved Ronald Reagan's life when he was at death's door.

A few hours after surgery, President McKinley was awake and was transferred via electric ambulance to the home of a local dignitary. He then waited for army nurses to arrive and provide post-operative care. Once again, he did not go to a modern hospital, but to a private home in Buffalo.

Over the next few days, the president seemed to rally; he was awake and conversational. Doctors were optimistic, so much so that on September 9, Vice President Teddy Roosevelt left his vigil at McKinley's bedside and returned to the Adirondacks to continue his interrupted family vacation.

McKinley then began to do poorly. He should have been

transferred to a hospital, but he wasn't. There had been three opportunities to care for McKinley in hospital; immediately after the shooting, immediately post operatively, and when McKinley began to do poorly.

Post-operative care at a private home was acceptable only if the patient was doing well. The president did not improve; he became sicker and started to fade. Gangrene, the result of bacterial infection, grew along the path of the bullet. By the morning of September 13, it was apparent that the president would not survive.

VP Teddy Roosevelt and family were camping just below the summit of Mt. Marcy, at 5,344 feet above sea level, the highest mountain in the Adirondacks. A runner came up the mountain and delivered a telegram to Roosevelt telling of McKinley's imminent death. He was being summoned to return to Buffalo from the Adirondacks.

At midnight, Vice President Roosevelt began a wild ride, racing down Mount Marcy at breakneck speed, in the dark of night, through the forested wilderness, in the pouring rain, using a relay team of three horses, buckboards and drivers to speed him forty miles over rough mountain roads to the railhead at North Creek, where he arrived at 4:46 a.m.[8]

But at 2:15 that same morning, President McKinley died. At that moment, somewhere during that wild ride down the mountain, TR automatically became the new president, an appropriate start for his presidency. That mountainside location has since been memorialized by a bronze marker set in granite blocks.

A special train then took TR to Albany, where another special train carried him to Buffalo, where he was sworn in as the twenty-sixth president of the United States at 3:32 p.m. on September 14, 1901. At forty-two years old, Theodore Roosevelt became the youngest president in US history. No one else has become president under circumstances like this.

McKinley's autopsy showed gangrene of the anterior and

posterior walls of the stomach. There was pancreatic necrosis with release of pancreatic fluids into the peritoneal cavity. There was also evidence of surgical wound infection that might have caused the gangrene. Before its completion, the autopsy was stopped by Mrs. McKinley, and so no final diagnosis was made.

But the autopsy did reveal a surgical wound infection that might have been caused by the failure to utilize full asepsis in the first aid station. Apparently, the surgeons did not wear gloves, used no disinfection, and used non-sterile probes. They also failed to drain the wound.[9]

A bizarre postmortem to the McKinley shooting occurred. Several weeks after McKinley's death, a young woman deliberately shot herself with the same caliber gun from the same distance with the same trajectory into her abdomen. Apparently looking for her fifteen minutes of fame, she essentially replicated McKinley's wound.

But Roswell Park was her physician and she had surgery in a hospital. Dr. Park made use of surgical retractors and electric lights. Unlike the president's doctors, Dr. Park used aseptic technique and drained the abdomen. She had the best possible care, was younger, and survived.[10] McKinley had *less than best* care, was older, and died.

11

PRESIDENTIAL COVER-UPS; PRIVACY AND ASSORTED SINS AND MISDEMEANORS

Following the three-ring circus that accompanied Garfield's shooting in 1881, presidents began to cover up their medical care in order to protect their privacy. Public humiliation seemed like too high a price to pay for being president. This chapter deals with the cover-ups of Chester Arthur and Grover Cleveland.

Before becoming Garfield's vice president, Chester Arthur had been one of the least attractive players in American politics. He had been the creature of Roscoe Conkling, the corrupt boss of the New York Republican Party. Arthur became collector of the Port of New York, the source of much of the money that fed corrupt state and national political activity. Somehow, he left the position without further tarnishing his already low reputation.

Before the 1880 election, Arthur had been Garfield's political enemy. However, after Garfield's election, Arthur became his dutiful VP and was loyal to Garfield and his policies. Recall Garfield's assassin shouting, "Hurrah! Arthur is President!"

Any premature assumption of power by VP Arthur might seem like the completion of a coup. Accordingly, after the shooting, Arthur remained a strict protector of Garfield and made no attempt to take over the presidency. This was despite the severity of Garfield's wounds, and the episodic confusion and delirium that accompanied his final days.

When Arthur became president in September 1881, he had a metamorphosis.[1] This creature of party politics and the spoils system became a strong supporter of civil service reform and cut himself off from any further dealings with Conkling. He would go on to create the first Civil Service Commission.

The death of Garfield had not only exposed the ignorance and medical malpractice of Dr. Bliss and his cohorts, but also exposed several flaws in the US electoral process. There were no provisions to provide relief for an ailing and disabled President Garfield as the 25th Amendment did not appear until 1967.

In October 1882, President Arthur was examined by the Surgeon General and was found to have *Bright's disease,* chronic *glomerulonephritis,* a serious inflammatory disease of the kidneys.[2] This diagnosis was confirmed by other physicians, but Arthur did not make this information public. Arthur's administration was the first to systematically cover up and lie to the public about a president's illness. Arthur wanted to protect his family from the humiliation suffered by the Garfields, and he succeeded.

A report about Arthur's illness was printed in the *New York Herald* but was emphatically denied by the administration. A close friend was trotted out who claimed "the president had malaria and was now recovering." President Arthur's official spokesman stated, "the president is in excellent health. Reports that he has *Bright's* disease are pure fiction." During the 1960 presidential campaign, Robert Kennedy would tell similar lies to the public about his brother, John, including a reference to non-existent malaria, an obvious attempt at obfuscation.

The *New York Tribune* wrote in October 1882, "I have it on the authority of the president himself that he is not troubled by Bright's disease or any other kidney complications." And that became the standard of presidential health bulletins until Eisenhower's heart attack in 1955.

Were Arthur's denials justified? He continued to serve as president even although he was terminally sick. He spared an already traumatized nation from another presidential health crisis. Recall that James Garfield had lingered for 11 weeks in 1881 as the national press conducted their lurid display of the president's agony.

Arthur prevented the spectacle of newspaper accounts about his illness by lying on several occasions to maintain the cover-up. He repeatedly made public declarations that he was in good health. During a rail road trip to Florida in 1883, he came close to death when a broken coupling side-railed his rail car for two hours in the blistering heat. Too bad that railroad air conditioning wasn't available in 1883, since the outdoors temperature during Arthur's trip was as high as 99 degrees F.

By showing up for work, staying alive, and averting a political crisis, Arthur performed a great service to the nation, validating Woody Allen's statement that "eighty percent of success is just showing up." Thankfully, Arthur lived to finish out Garfield's four-year term and was succeeded as president in March 1885 by Grover Cleveland. The new Succession Act of 1886 provided some remedies for the problems of vacancies in the line of succession.

Succeeding presidents expanded the reasons for presidential cover-ups to include protecting the public from traumatic political events, hiding medical incompetence and presidential disability, allowing for political usurpation to occur, and shielding various machinations, crimes, and misdemeanors.

All the following presidents and/or their doctors participated in medical cover-ups, and most of them lied about what they had done. Included are the reasons (excuses) for the cover-ups.

. . .

REASONS for the Cover-up (they all involved the health of the president):

- **Arthur:** To spare the nation and his family from another presidential health crisis.
- **Cleveland:** To spare the nation from a worsening of the Panic of 1893.
- **Wilson:** To hide the political usurpation by Mrs. Wilson.
- **FDR:** To protect multiple beneficiaries; hide Dr. McIntire's "incompetence;" protect Democratic politicos; protect the Allied war effort; protect FDR from his many political opponents.
- **JFK:** To maintain the image of vigor; keep hidden JFK's many ailments and his use of amphetamines.
- **Ike:** To hide Dr. Snyder's initial failure to diagnose a heart attack

Note the overlap of secrecy, incompetence, and disability that occurred among these men. Neither the public nor the presidents were well served during these areas of overlap.[3] The veil of secrecy was finally lifted by Eisenhower and Reagan, who both received excellent care, and were never disabled, despite severe disease and injury. Wilson, FDR, and JFK all took part in cover-ups that had serious consequences for the nation and the world. Our book will devote at least one chapter to each of them.

As news broadcasting has evolved to a 24-hour cycle, public figures find it difficult to maintain any semblance of privacy. Some observers believe that the president can have little expectation of privacy, but that presidential candidates should expect some more privacy.

Hopefully, the twenty-fifth Amendment will be a political remedy for future incidents of presidential incapacity due to illness and surgery. Doctors are not now involved in the political process, nor should they be. The public should be notified whenever the president is on the cusp of disability or has a disabling disease.[4]

GROVER CLEVELAND UNDERWENT a secret surgical operation that took him and the nation to a very dangerous place—the narrow and difficult to navigate East River in New York City. He had incompetent care, but the cover-up was so spectacular it is included in this section on cover-ups.

It was the efficient system of the aseptic modern operating room illuminated with electric lights, that we saw in the Dr. Agnew painting that led to better outcomes for patients. The following sounds unbelievable but is true. American surgeons would abandon the hospital operating room and trained surgical teams to perform surgery on the president on a yacht that cruised up the ever-treacherous East River of New York City.

It was 1893 and the recent memory of Garfield may have provided a reason to avoid repeating the public spectacle of a sick president. But isn't having secret surgery on a moving boat going "overboard?"

Cleveland's doctors did not lack confidence. In their zeal, they rushed to surgery, which they botched and put the president of the United States in a very dangerous place, on a moving boat, under ether anesthesia,

A political/economic crisis led to this incredible event. After the Civil War, the United States had based its currency on silver deposits in the West. This was formulated in the Sherman Silver Act which favored small farmers, debtors, and working people. But in 1893, the US economy tanked. Wall Street collapsed, railroads went bankrupt, and European bondholders were calling their notes. The Panic of 1893 was second only to the economic collapse of 1929. Cleveland felt he had to repeal the Sherman Silver Act to end the Panic.

Grover Cleveland was inaugurated in March of 1893, and within a few days he noticed a rough spot on his *palate*. The White House doctor thought it to be a *sarcoma*, a form of cancer. Samples of the lesion were taken and sent to pathologists at the Armed Forces Institute of Pathology. They felt that the evaluation of the samples were inconclusive, although suggestive of *carcinoma*, another type of cancer. This was not surprising, since Cleveland had been a heavy cigar smoker. The tumor was also referred to as an *epithelioma*, which is nonspecific for a new growth of epithelial origin. That could be either benign or malignant. At best, there was a consensus formed to remove the probably malignant tumor.

Despite the lack of a definitive diagnosis, Cleveland's doctors arranged for radical resection of his jaw, an operation that in hospital had a fourteen percent mortality rate. It was a dangerous operation, but Cleveland demanded that all his care be done in secret.[5] His reasoning was as follows: "News that the president had cancer would further worsen the Panic and cripple the president politically. The surgery had to be kept secret so as not to worsen public anxiety." Cleveland's VP, Adlai Stevenson, Sr., supported the Sherman Act, and so Cleveland did not confide in him and kept him out of the loop, including the plans for surgery.

Cleveland and his good friend and personal physician, Dr. Joseph Bryant of New York, organized the plan to perform the secret surgery on the private steam yacht *Oneida* as it cruised up the East River. Bryant assembled a dream team of surgeons to assist him with the operation. His first recruit was Dr. William Keen, who was the first American surgeon to remove a brain tumor.

Bryant also oversaw preparations on the *Oneida*, anchored in the East River. The yacht's small, dark saloon was transformed into a makeshift operating room. Here the president would sit for the operation, as there was no operating table. The only artificial light would come from a single electric bulb connected to a portable battery. The larger pieces of equipment, including tanks of oxygen and nitrous oxide, were quietly delivered to the yacht.

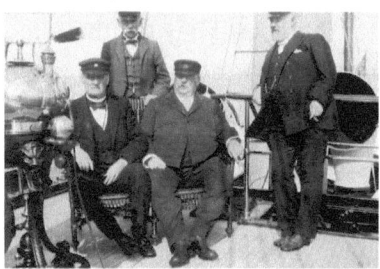

Image 12: An obese Grover Cleveland, seated in middle of the photo, awaits surgery on board the Oneida. *1893*

Operating in a small, dimly lit, and poorly ventilated space on a moving boat appeared to place unnecessary extra risks to an already high-risk procedure. In the vernacular of the times, if anything went wrong, Cleveland's doctors would be up to the "hub in mud." As the yacht set sail, Dr. Bryant called out to the captain, "If you hit a rock, hit it good and hard so that we will all go to the bottom." Apparently, the doctors were aware of the risks they were taking.

There were many problems associated with this hastily arranged surgery performed on President Cleveland on a sailing yacht.

1. **Dangerous surgery.** The risks were enormous, the benefits dubious. The fourteen percent hospital mortality for this surgery would almost certainly be greater on a yacht.

2. **A ship at sea** has at least six types of motion, including up and down of the bow, twisting of the bow, side-to-side motion of the ship, bow to stern, stern to bow motion, and forward motion of the ship. That makes the plane of the opera-

tive field unstable. Now add in the East River with its ever-changing tidal currents, and the surgical risk becomes high.

3. Unfamiliar team. The surgical team assembled on the *Oneida* had never worked together; in fact most of them had never met before. None of them had ever performed surgery on a boat, let alone one that was cruising up the East River.

4. Poor preparations done in haste. Cleveland had breakfast before the surgery, which is usually not allowed pre-operatively because of the risk of *aspiration* of food. In case the patient vomits, you don't want a stomach full of food to enter the lungs and cause pneumonia.

The surgeons were prepared to use electrocautery, even though the ether anesthesia that was eventually used was explosive. The smallest spark could set it off. How could the president, or for that matter any patient, have been placed at such risk? The whole aim of pre-operative care is to reduce the risk for the patient. What could possibly be the reasons for such poor judgment?

The standard of care will provide for the best outcome, for every one rich or poor, black or white. There should be no special accommodations made for special people. Expediency does not guarantee a good outcome. Appeals to the vanity of doctors and patients that the patients are special people who require special rules frequently cause problems. There should never be any political considerations in planning for surgery. In addition, is it ever a good idea to have your surgeon be a close friend? Remember Dr. Craik and George Washington.

5. What is wrong with this picture? The surgery began on July 1, 1893, with the very obese Cleveland strapped upright in a chair lashed against the mast.[6] Remember that hospitals had been open for business in the US since 1736.

6. Failure of surgery. Nitrous oxide anesthesia was initially used, but it soon became apparent that it was wearing off. Ether anesthesia became necessary. The surgeons did resort to electrocautery during surgery, and fortunately there was no explosion.

∼

THE PRESIDENCY once again survived a great threat. There were, however, several surgical complications. Cleveland began to bleed, and the operation took much longer than anticipated. At the end of the operation the doctors found that much of the tumor had not been resected.[7] Expediency and secrecy had not made for a good medical/surgical outcome.

So on July 17, 1893, a second operation to remove any residual tumor was performed on the *Oneida*, with most of the original cast of characters. Not much is known about that second surgery, except that it was apparently successful. However, the president again was unnecessarily placed at high risk, as in-hospital surgery would have been safer. The cover-up was still in play.[8]

News of the July 1 surgery was leaked to several newspapers by Dr. Ferdinand Hasbrouck, the dentist who removed some teeth to facilitate removal of the tumor. But this leak was quashed by a well-organized cover-up that began before surgery with the pre-operative announcement that Cleveland was on the yacht for a vacation and that the dentist had been on board only for routine dental work.

After the second surgery, the president was fitted with an oral rubber jaw prosthesis that was placed inside his mouth and *hid* the operative defect from view. Since surgery had been done inside the mouth with no external incisions, there were no visible signs of surgery. The public appearances of the president supported his contention that he did not have cancer. Cleveland looked to be in good health and spoke with his usual normal voice. There was no apparent change to his face and his familiar walrus mustache appeared unchanged. Friendly newspapers portrayed Cleveland as healthy. The public remained completely in the dark.[9]

The risky surgery was in vain. The Silver Act was repealed, but the Panic and financial depression continued. The surgery remained a well-kept secret, until 1917.

IN 1967, the surgical specimen from Cleveland's tumor was reviewed and found to be a *verrucous* (wart like) carcinoma, a slow growing indolent tumor usually treated with only local excision. This implies that the radical surgery had been unnecessary.

Even that opinion and diagnosis is questionable, however, because Cleveland had an extensive tumor that went from the roots of his teeth to just below his maxillary sinus. Maybe the extensive surgery was necessary? Today, over a hundred years after Cleveland's surgery, there is still uncertainty surrounding the exact details of the pathological diagnosis, with four different diagnoses offered to the public: sarcoma, carcinoma, epithelioma, or verrucous carcinoma.

The Cleveland cover-up had been justified as a means of lessening the Panic of 1893, and to hide the radical care given to the president. But the secrecy had also served a second purpose: to cover-up the risks taken by Cleveland's surgeons and the failure of the first surgery. No matter how eminent they were, they unnecessarily put their patient's life at great risk and repeated that risk with a second operation.

What were the doctors thinking?[10]

12

BENEFITS OF HOSPITALIZATION

By the end of the American Civil War, hospitals were becoming the only acceptable place to treat seriously ill patients. The concentration of medical talent, the presence of nurses, abundant supplies, sterile instruments, and clean, well-ventilated settings, all provided a better outcome for patients.

One cringes upon learning that Presidents Garfield, Cleveland, and McKinley were not treated in hospitals but in private homes, train stations, exhibition halls, and on a yacht sailing up the East River. Furthermore, Garfield died at a seaside home and McKinley died in a private home in Buffalo, NY.

Future presidents would not fare much better. Wilson was treated for a small stroke on a moving train; Harding was treated for complex cardiac disease in a hotel room. In 1974, Nixon may have been treated for thrombophlebitis on an airplane en route to the Middle East, and shortly thereafter on an airplane trip to the USSR.

The decision makers for these presidents were behind the times and did not take advantage of the many improvements and benefits of hospital care. Avoidance of hospitalization made some sense in 1781, but not in 1881, 1901, 1919, 1923, or 1974.

For much of history, hospitals had been fearful places, best exemplified by the horror of obstetrical care in Vienna in the mid-19th century. Women who gave birth on the university obstetrical wards in the capital cities of Europe had a much higher death rate than those who delivered at home, as much as seventeen times higher.[1]

The usual cause of maternal death was puerperal fever due to streptococcal infection acquired during childbirth. But progress came, beginning with Semmelweis whose words were not silenced even when he was in a lunatic asylum. His solution was pretty simple, obstetrical staff needed to wash their hands before examining patients.[2]

During the Crimean War of 1853-1856, Florence Nightingale greatly reduced the death rate of British soldiers in her hospital at Scutari from 42 percent to an incredible 2 percent. She did this by initiating some basic sanitary reforms, ritual hand-washing techniques, cleaning latrines, flushing out sewers, reducing overcrowding, and improving the ventilation of hospital wards.[3]

At the onset of the American Civil War, thousands of Union soldiers. were hospitalized under awful conditions, and the hospitals were described as slaughterhouses. As the war continued, health care personnel improved their skills at the postgraduate school of OJT, on the job training. The best surgeons were eventually identified and selected to be the ones who did most of the major surgery. For example, only one in fifteen physicians were authorized to do amputations. The others assisted, triaged, did minor surgery, changed dressings, etc. Necessity had led to surgical specialization.

After Gettysburg, the Union wounded were retrieved from the battlefield and taken to hospital no later than 12 hours after combat. Teams of dedicated drivers, horses and wagons were assembled, and the ambulance corps was formed. Getting the wounded to hospital as fast as possible became an important part of care.

About 15,000 women, working for the US Sanitary Commission, came to volunteer for the Union Army. Among these women were Clara Barton and Dorothy Dix. Another notable Civil War nurse was Walt Whitman who served more than 600 tours of duty. They assisted with surgery, worked as nurses on the hospital wards, and administered hospital ships.

Hospitals wards became large well-lit, well-ventilated rooms, that were forever being mopped clean. Frequently there was a breezy sun parlor at one end for convalescent patients.

Professional staff were supplemented by volunteers who would bring the comforts of home to the bedside, writing letters, bringing books and newspapers, etc. This was the legacy of Florence Nightingale.[4]

Medical and Surgical Advances during the American Civil War [5]

- Use of quinine for the prevention of malaria
- Use of quarantine to eliminate Yellow Fever
- Successful treatment of gangrene with bromine and isolation
- Development of an ambulance system
- Use of trains and steamships to transport patients
- Development of large general hospitals
- Creation of specialty surgery and hospitals
- Safe use of anesthetics
- Rudimentary neuro surgery
- Demonstrated techniques for arterial ligation
- First performance of plastic surgery

The result of these changes was seen during the last year of the war, when the in-hospital death rate in Union Army hospitals fell to 8 percent. Similarly, the death rate was 9 percent at the large Confederate hospital in Richmond.[6]

The reforms and changes continued after the war with attention to personal hygiene, generalized cleanliness, growth of professional nursing, and well-ventilated hospital wards.

British and American civilian hospitals adopted these measures and in-hospital survival rates improved dramatically.

Lister's antiseptic techniques using carbolic acid to sterilize the skin had made slow inroads due to the failure of others to reproduce his results. Few people could recreate his mindset of absolute zero tolerance. Carbolic acid was irritating to the skin. Over several years, antisepsis evolved to asepsis, with washing hands with soap and water before surgery, with sterile drapes and gowns, gloves, instruments, and masks. There was to be no more carbolic acid in surgery. These benefits were easier to duplicate and were rapidly adopted worldwide.

1873. Johns Hopkins medical school was founded, and along with it came the birth of the American academic research medical center that would come to rival any others in the world.

1876. The centennial year is an interesting dividing point in American history. Two events highlight the two sides of the Centennial divide.

1. Custer's Last Stand took place in June 1876, marking the end of the first century of the Republic.
2. In Baltimore September 1876, the British scientist Thomas Huxley[7] delivered the opening address at the inaugural ceremony for Johns Hopkins University. This was a marker for the beginning of the second century of the Republic.

The US now began a new chapter in its rise to the scientific leadership of the modern world.

1876 Lister toured the US, preaching the benefits of antisepsis.

1889 Johns Hopkins Hospital opened and reinvented the hospital.

The accomplishments of Drs. Welch, Osler, Kelly, and Halstead, the "Big Four" at Hopkins would change the medical world.[8] Their images can be seen on the front cover in the painting by John Singer Sargent. Two of them, Osler and Welch, had trained with Rudolf Virchow in Berlin, another example of trans-Atlantic exchange of scientific information.[9]

Dr. William Welch, the pathologist, was the first on board and he recruited the other three to Hopkins. Welch was responsible for training many outstanding physicians of the day, including Walter Reed and Simon Flexner, first president of the Rockefeller Institute.

Dr. William Osler, the first chief of the Department of Medicine, is credited with originating the idea of a residency, where recently graduated doctors received advanced training while treating patients under supervision. He introduced the idea of bringing medical students into areas of actual patient care. His textbook of medicine became the standard reference in the English-speaking world. Osler's other contributions to medical education included the creation of "grand rounds," with staff physicians discussing the most difficult cases in front of assembled medical students.

Dr. Howard Kelly is credited with establishing gynecology as a unique bona fide specialty. He invented numerous medical devices, including a urinary cystoscope. He was one of the first to use radium to treat cancer, and apparently received his initial supply of the radioactive element directly from Madame Curie.

Dr. William Halsted, the first chief of the Department of Surgery, established the modern surgical principles for the control of bleeding, accurate surgical anatomical dissection, and complete sterility of the operating theater. He performed the world's first radical mastectomy for breast cancer. Halsted also established the first formal surgical residency training program in the US. He was the first prominent surgeon to wear surgical gloves, and that is part of a love story.

Caroline Hampton, a member of a prominent southern family, entered nursing school in New York City, graduating in 1888. In 1889, she moved to Baltimore and it was here that she met Halsted. She was appointed chief nurse to Halsted and before long the two became romantically involved. Halsted had decided to use a combination of carbolic acid and mercuric chloride as a disinfectant during his surgical procedures.

Hampton, acting as his scrub nurse, handled these chemicals regularly and as a consequence developed severe contact dermatitis on her hands. Halsted reached out to the Goodyear Rubber Co. to create a rubber glove that she could wear during surgery to protect her hands.[10]

These proved to be so satisfactory that additional gloves were ordered for other staff members, including Halstead. Before long, other operating staff and surgeons began wearing gloves to protect their hands and in time their use became commonplace. But the major consequence was an unexpected benefit. Wearing surgical gloves decreased the incidence of postoperative infections from seventeen percent to two percent.[11]

Sterilized surgical rubber gloves were introduced in 1894 and by the early 1900s all surgeons were wearing sterilized gloves. The "Big Four" had reinvented the hospital.[12]

Electric lighting became readily available after 1879 and, accordingly, the modern hospital was brighter. Thanks to Florence Nightingale, it would also be better ventilated and cleaner. Nurses brought a duty of care to the hospital. They were professionals, products of nursing schools all across the land. Many were dedicated middle and upper-class women, and their presence greatly improved patient comfort and care.

The germ theory was universally accepted, and the aseptic technique prevailed. Hospitals used sterile supplies and instruments that were readily available on site. They became a place of restoration of health, of successful surgery, a model of the achievements of modern science. There was a concentration of medical talent in the great hospitals across the nation, an intellectual fervor, and dedication to research and teaching,

Among the best known hospitals were Mount Sinai, Cleveland Clinic, Mayo Clinic, Barnes Hospital, Massachusetts General, Johns Hopkins, Columbia Presbyterian, and Stanford. The learning curve was moving forward, and medical care greatly improved all across the nation.

The failure to hospitalize Garfield, Cleveland, McKinley, Wilson, Harding, and Nixon boggles the mind, and is so incredible, that the most bizarre conspiratorial theories sound plausible in comparison. What would be the benefit of going to the hospital for each of them?

For interest sakes, let's also include Lincoln, whose hospitalization would have been in vain in 1865. At the time there were no neurosurgeons and no neurosurgical instruments. Modern neurosurgery in the US would only begin in 1888 with William Keen, and only in 1901 with Harvey Cushing did it truly blossom.

Let's go back to Garfield. If his wound was surgically explored in hospital under anesthesia, using sterile techniques, his outcome might have been different. Remember the death rate for inpatients in 1865 in Union Army hospitals was only 8 percent, and many patients were soldiers recovering from gunshot wounds.

Garfield was shot and surgically probed while lying on the floor of a train station. This was 1881, not 1781, and it was a very disturbing moment in US history. A hospital in 1881 would probably be clean, well lit, well ventilated, and equipped with appropriate supplies and staff.

You would expect none of that to be present in a train station. In hospital, casual passers-by might be restrained from poking their finger into a patient's wound. In hospital, you would expect to find nurses protecting their patients. The best thing for Garfield would have been to give him some pain medicine and get him off the floor and out of the train station and into a hospital. Do nothing else, no probing and no surgery.

Grover Cleveland had surgery on a boat traveling up the East River to maintain secrecy and not upset the financial markets with news of his cancer. His surgeons had rushed to surgery and put him at extraordinary risk for dubious political reasons. The various motions of the boat could not have led to a stable operative field.

In hospital, more time could be made available to do surgery under more favorable conditions, perhaps doing the entire surgery in one sitting, and not subjecting him to the risks of a second operation. Cleveland had sacrificed his chance of receiving good care in vain because the Panic of 1893 continued.

William McKinley was shot in 1901 and treated in a makeshift first aid room on the grounds of an exhibition. He would have been better served in a well-equipped modern hospital, with electric lights, surgical retractors, and X-ray machines. A bonus would have been the presence of the expert surgeon Dr. Roswell Park at the Buffalo General Hospital.

An exhausted Woodrow Wilson probably had a small stroke, or *transient cerebral ischemia*, in September 25, 1919, in Pueblo, Colorado. After a brief period of time, he recovered completely. There are other diagnostic possibilities, but the truth remains unknown since all his medical records are missing. He did not go to a local hospital but returned to Washington DC. Shortly afterwards, on October 2, he had a massive stroke, resulting in permanent paralysis.

Hospitalization in Pueblo would have offered Wilson a much-needed respite from his barnstorming tour across the US of 8,000 miles in 22 days. It would have saved him an immediate 1,651-mile return train trip to DC. He could have been sedated, placed on a low salt diet, and rested while he recovered.

In hospital, there would be equipment to evaluate his cardiovascular system: EKG technology had been available since 1905; chest X-ray machines had been in general use since 1900; and blood pressure measurement was generally available in the US since 1901. Maybe the use of these instruments could have prevented the stroke that he suffered on October 2, 1919.

It was surprising that Wilson was not hospitalized following his October 2 stroke. His physician Dr. Cary Grayson had trained with William Osler at Johns Hopkins, the epicenter of great hospital care.

Following his October stroke, Wilson had an episode of acute urinary retention. A local Washington urologist came to the White House but was unable to place a catheter in Wilson's bladder. The procedure of bladder catheterization might have been more successful in hospital with trained assistants, a well-supplied procedure room, and better illumination. The president suffered in agony for several days until his urine finally passed spontaneously.[16]

No patient should be allowed to suffer like that. Return with different sized catheters or have someone else try the procedure. Certainly no one who just had a stroke should be made to strain attempting to urinate. Once again, the president's doctors were not being strong advocates for their patients.

The death of President Warren Harding in a hotel room highlights the folly of the failure to hospitalize him and demonstrated a lack of judgment by his physicians. It also displayed timidity and failure to advocate for a famous patient. This failure to provide in-hospital care for Harding is extraordinary. One factor leading to Harding's incompetent care was that he had too many doctors. The group-think had descended to the lowest common denominator and followed the lead of the least competent physician among them.

Harding was fifty-seven years old when he died in 1923. For the past several years, he was known to have systolic hypertension, and sugar in his urine (a sign of diabetes), both diseases having a predilection for coronary disease. Since 1918, he had suffered from shortness of breath, bouts of chest pain, and difficulty sleeping unless his head was propped up on several pillows. These were symptoms of coronary disease and/or congestive heart failure, but apparently that diagnosis was not made prior to his death.

On June, 20, 1923, Harding traveled by train from Washington DC to St. Louis where he gave one of the first presidential speeches to be broadcast live by radio. We are now in modern times.

The train then continued to the West Coast where Harding began a fateful trip to Alaska aboard the USS *Henderson*. On July 27, he became ill with cramps, indigestion, fever, and distressing shortness of breath. The president chalked this up to "food poisoning" and the stresses of being on a 15,000 mile cross-country speaking tour.

Mr. and Mrs. Harding's favorite doctor, a *homeopathic* physician from Ohio named Charles Sawyer, was with the presidential entourage. Dr. Sawyer said Harding was sick from having eaten tainted crabmeat. That was not likely, since no one else in the party had food poisoning. Harding probably never had any crabmeat on the trip; apparently, crabmeat was never on the menu. Yet, this story of tainted crab meat still continues in circulation.

Two other doctors in the group, Dr. Boone and Dr. Work, examined Harding and found that he had an enlarged heart with elevated blood pressure. This was good evidence that Harding was suffering from heart disease.[14] Dr. Sawyer insisted that Harding only had indigestion.

Herbert Hoover, who was part of the presidential party, arranged for the group to go immediately to San Francisco where they were met by Dr. Charles Cooper, a cardiologist, and Dr. Ray Wilbur, former dean of Stanford Medical School. There were now five doctors on the medical team.

Harding was taken to a room in the Palace Hotel in San

Francisco rather than to a modern hospital, the new San Francisco General Hospital that opened in 1915. The reasoning behind this decision remains obscure. Maybe Harding was suicidal as several authors have suggested, and he refused hospitalization on that basis. But now the doctors knew Harding had a large heart and was short of breath. To repeat, that is congestive heart failure until proven otherwise.

Why didn't the doctor's insist that Harding go to a hospital? They knew that Harding had heart failure and suspected he had a heart attack but failed to state that publicly. The failure to be strong independent advocates for the presidential patient is a recurrent theme in our story. Expediency and political considerations too often trumped advocacy. That usually results in dire consequences for patient and sometimes the nation. The medical group had descended to the level of its most incompetent member.

It is proper once again to mention our timeline. We are no longer in the Dark Ages; Harding's radio broadcast was a marker of modern times. Modern hospitals and medical centers were operating. Chest X-ray and EKG were readily available.

But for Harding's final days, it was as though he fell down a rabbit hole and became a time traveler. He was being treated in a hotel room, which was the standard of care in 660 C.E. when the Hôtel-Dieu opened for business as a plague house in Paris.

Dr. Wilbur obtained a medical history of pain in Harding's chest that radiated down both arms, especially the left arm. Didn't that sound like coronary disease? Why didn't Dr. Cooper, the cardiologist, perform an EKG, technology invented in 1905 and readily available in 1923?

Since 1910, Dr. Robert Herrick had been advancing the idea that myocardial infarction (MI) was a common clinical condition of living humans and not a postmortem effect. This finally gained consensus among American doctors, and by 1921, myocardial infarction was the number one cause of death on US death certificates.[15]

The signs and symptoms of MI were well known to practicing physicians, and it was and still is relatively easy to make the diagnosis with an EKG. The failure to do an EKG during Harding's final illness was just extraordinary. How can you possibly explain that?

The most critical error was taking the president to a hotel room, and not to a hospital. What were they all thinking? The doctors, except for Sawyer, were well trained and previously competent. The Palace Hotel did not advertise itself as an acute care hospital. Most important, EKG machines were not usually found there or in any hotel.

The next day, Harding had a fever of 102 degrees F and was diagnosed with pneumonia, prompting the cancellation of his remaining California appearances. An X-ray appeared that had been taken a few days before (on board the ship?) and it showed pneumonia. But that did not give the doctors current information whether the pneumonia was getting better or worse.

X-rays need to be dated to allow the doctors to match the findings on the chest X-ray with the patient's clinical condition on that same date. That helps determine whether the patient is worsening or improving. It would have been very helpful to repeat the chest X-ray, but this also was not available at the Palace Hotel.

Oxygen therapy would have been helpful for either pneumonia, heart failure and/or heart attack, but it was not used. To restate the obvious, EKG, chest X-ray, and oxygen therapy are not usually available in hotels, but are usually found in hospitals, where Harding needed to be.

On August 1, his temperature was back to normal, his lungs were clearing up, and he was capable of sitting up in bed, reading, and eating solid food. Harding was given digitalis, and he improved over the next day. That therapeutic response suggested the presence of congestive heart failure that was being treated.

Dr. Sawyer decided August 2 would be a good time to go on vacation. Why would he do that? Unfortunately, for Harding's life and Sawyer's reputation, Harding died suddenly the next day, August 3. There is no agreed upon version of the events of that day such as who was in the room when he died or what time he died.

The importance of the French school is again noted, keeping records is so critical, especially in a rapidly changing situation. There are at least three different versions of what happened that day. The failure to keep a record of Harding's illness could be due to incompetence, in-difference, expediency, or participation in a cover-up for whatever reason. We can only guess.

Dr. Sawyer said that the cause of death was a cerebral hemorrhage. The four other doctors disagreed. They all conferred and signed a joint statement stating the cause of death was *apoplexy*, an archaic term for a stroke. But there was no evidence to support that.

Col. Edmund Starling, senior Secret Service agent on site, suspected foul play which, in itself, was pretty extraordinary. He separately interviewed all the doctors who had signed the apoplexy statement. Each of them told him that the apoplexy was the cause of death. Harding's wife refused to permit an autopsy, and that ended any further investigation.

Today, most historians accept that Harding died from a heart attack and/or congestive heart failure, either one worsened by a recent bout of pneumonia. The failure to send Harding to a hospital highlights the folly of this group of doctors attempting to treat the president in a hotel room. At the final moment they were more concerned about showing professional courtesy for Dr. Sawyer than for being advocates for their patient.

Similar to the experience of Garfield, this was another

example of the failure of team medicine and the ease of finding the lowest common denominator of medical care. *Facilis descensus Averno.* Easy is the way down to Hell.

The incomplete and inconsistent documentation of events, especially in a hotel room, gives credence to the tale that Harding was poisoned, a tale that still circulates years later. There is still no plausible explanation of how Harding wound up being treated in a hotel room.

Not going to the general hospital shields the president from publicity, offers him some privacy, avoids embarrassment or need to explain his medical condition. It appeals to president's vanity and need for a la carte VIP service. Expediency and cutting corners may be seen as premium service for the elite. But there is always a price to pay and Harding paid with his life.

13

PANDEMICS: WILSON AND TRUMP, LESSONS NOT LEARNED

There have been two deadly pandemics in recent memory, the 1918 Influenza pandemic and the 2020 Covid 19 pandemic. They are similar in many ways and many of the same lessons apply. Unfortunately, many of the lessons of 1918 apparently were forgotten, or dismissed, as the same mistakes were repeated and hundreds of thousands died needlessly in 2020–2022.

Before we talk about Wilson's stroke and cover-up let's review the Influenza epidemic of 1918–1919, because that was when things began to go wrong for Wilson.

Woodrow Wilson was re-elected president in 1916 by a narrow margin, 277 to 254 electoral votes. He campaigned on a slogan of "he kept us out of war." One month into his second term, he asked Congress to declare war against Germany and Austria. The halcyon days of pre-war America, with its special intimacy of personal relations, would soon be replaced by the anomie, chaos, and violence of World War I and pandemic.[1]

Influenza is an acute viral illness that effects the respiratory system with a clinical spectrum ranging from mild upper respiratory infection (most common) to fatal pneumonia. It is spread from person to person by respiratory droplets and is very contagious.[2] Influenza pandemics occurred in cycles of about twenty years or so. Recovery from influenza gives immunity only to that particular strain of the virus in circulation at the time.

Wilson was intimately involved with the Influenza epidemic, both as a patient and as a passive presidential observer who did and said nothing to support his countrymen who were dying by the thousands. His dereliction of duty enhanced the global spread of the disease and led to the deaths of millions. No other president helped spread an epidemic as did Wilson.

Wilson's failure to defend the nation from Influenza in 1918 was equivalent to Buchanan's failure to defend the Union from secession in 1860–1861. Trump's failure to take leadership of the Covid 19 pandemic of 2020 completes the trio of presidents who failed to successfully defend the nation during a time of crisis.

THE GREAT INFLUENZA Pandemic of 1918 occurred in four waves:

1. March 1918, US Army training camps in the midwestern US
2. Autumn 1918, worldwide, a lethal mutation on the Western Front
3. Spring 1919, mainly in Europe; Wilson infected in Paris
4. Spring 1920, worldwide, minimal US involvement, milder disease

The first wave, in the spring of 1918, occurred mainly in US Army training camps.

The second wave was the deadliest. It began in the fall of

1918, simultaneously in Boston, Brest, France, and Freetown, Sierra Leone in west Africa. All three cities were major seaports for Allied troopships. By the end of the second wave, civilians were infected as frequently as the military as the disease spread to the soldiers' girlfriends, relatives, and neighbors, and to shipyard and railroad workers, etc.

There were a total over 400,000 Influenza deaths in Germany during the four waves, which was a slightly higher rate than in the US. There was also a higher rate of disease in the German Army. In March 1918, Germany launched its last-ditch military offensive, but it stalled because they began to run out of fighting men due to the epidemic. At the same time, the Americans were adding 250,000 men per month to the Allied army. All the armies were rife with the disease but the "Yanks kept coming" across the ocean to the battlefield. Germany finally ran out of men before the Allies did and asked for an armistice.

The third wave of influenza hit Europe in the spring of 1919, after the Armistice. The US was spared most of the third wave, but Germany was hit very hard as the wave coincided with the continuation of the Allied naval blockade of Germany which lasted until July 1919.

Wilson supported the food blockade and that led to famine and 500,000 deaths from starvation which were closely linked with the third influenza wave. Many German influenza deaths occurred in starving people, making it difficult to distinguish famine from influenza infection as the cause of death.

The fourth wave hit Europe in 1920, killing hundreds of thousands in Europe. The US again had a much lower rate.

The term "Spanish Flu" is a terrible misnomer. There was nothing particularly Spanish about the epidemic. Each of the warring nations had very strict newspaper censorship. Their governments believed that any news of the epidemic would benefit the enemy.[3] So, newspapers in the US, UK, France, Italy,

Germany, Austria, and Russia had no news of the pandemic. But since Spain was a neutral nation, its papers carried news about the pandemic along with news from Spain. Since the news of the Influenza pandemic originated in Spain, it became good policy for the various belligerent nations to refer to the pandemic as the Spanish Flu.

No nation wanted to claim responsibility for being the birth place of the pandemic. This was very important in an era of rampant nationalism. Similar events occurred with Covid 19 in 2020 as Trump kept referring to the pandemic as the China flu. This was a reflection of his America First policy and an attempt to deflect his failures onto the Chinese.

After the 1918 Armistice, the western strip of Germany was occupied by French troops, some of whom were soldiers from Morocco. That was seen as a racial affront by many Germans. Germany was suffering human misery to the nth degree—military defeat, foreign occupation, Influenza epidemic, political riots, famine, and death. The Versailles treaty forced Germany to accept the war guilt clause along with other punitive measures. It is easy to connect these dots along a single thread giving rise to Nazism.

PAST SOLUTIONS TO EPIDEMICS: During the smallpox pandemic of 1776, Washington employed quarantine and isolation to control the epidemic in Massachusetts. The local cholera epidemic in 1854 London ended when John Snow removed the handle from the water Broad Street pump. The 1904 Yellow Fever outbreak in Cuba ended when Dr. Gorgas covered the water barrels in Havana and reduced the Yellow Fever death rate to zero.[4]

All are simple and brilliant solutions. Recall from the American Revolution that an army on the move is a powerful vector for spreading disease, especially during an epidemic. Wilson could never quite grasp that concept.

From 1914 to 1918, Dr. William Gorgas had re-appeared on the scene, this time as surgeon general of the US Army. Could he repeat the success that he had with Yellow Fever, another viral disease? His plan to stop influenza from spreading was to halt the overseas troop shipments, because that was the vector for the Pandemic.

Unfortunately, neither Washington nor Jefferson nor Teddy Roosevelt were in office in 1918. Wilson was in office and although he was not yet demented, he did *not* have the *right stuff* to support Gorgas and stop the troop movements. Gorgas underwent mandatory retirement on October 4, 1918, at the peak of the second wave—an example of terrible timing.[5]

By 1918, the world had entered an era of enlightenment, invention, and great discovery.[6]

1879 Edison invented the incandescent light bulb
1885 Louis Pasteur created the rabies vaccine
1889 Johns Hopkins Hospital opened
1895 Diphtheria anti-toxin commercially available
1895 Roentgen discovered the Xray
1901 Rockefeller Institute was founded
1901 Marconi's first trans-Atlantic radio transmission
1903 Wright brothers flew at Kitty Hawk

THERE WAS high expectation that modern 20th century science could find a solution for the pandemic. The light microscope had become a magic lantern, illuminating many facets of the major infectious diseases, especially, the identification of offending bacterial organisms.

Scientists were looking hard but using an inadequate tool, the light microscope.[7] Unfortunately, Influenza is not caused by any bacteria, but by a virus, invisible under the light microscope. It was very disappointing that the light microscope and modern 1918 microbiology could not identify the causative agent of Influenza.

Nevertheless, Yellow Fever, smallpox, and rabies had been controlled despite the offending viruses never being seen. Vaccines were being made to control cholera, typhoid, diphtheria, and to protect against rattlesnake venom and tetanus. The not unreasonable hope was that similar success could be found for Influenza.

Unfortunately, that did not take place in the early 20th century. Viruses were not described until the late 19th century, and they were not *visualized* until after the introduction of the electron microscope in 1931.

THE SCOPE **of the Influenza Epidemic in 1918.** The population of the world in 1920 was about 1.86 billion people. Almost a billion people became infected, with 40 million deaths.[7] The pandemic occurred everywhere on earth except for American Samoa, which employed strict quarantine for several years. British Samoa, forty miles away did not, and about 20 percent of that population died from influenza. On American Samoa, the total deaths from influenza were zero. Once again, during the 2020 Covid 19 pandemic there have been zero deaths on American Samoa, which again employed strict quarantine. A few cases were brought to the island but were successfully quarantined. Strict quarantine saves lives.

In 1918, the US had a population of about 106 million, and about twenty million people became infected with about 675,000 deaths. That was more than the number of Americans killed in combat in World War I, World War II, Korea, and Vietnam combined (423,000). There is a consensus that the 675,000 number probably was an undercount for the deaths in the US.[8]

For example, who recorded the dead Native Americans?

The immigrant population was hard hit, and since many spoke no English, many of those deaths did not get properly recorded. In the slums of the big cities, the death carts would patrol the streets at night picking up the bodies left on the front porch or left in the street. Who recorded those deaths? Untold thousands were buried in mass graves, as communities ran out of coffins. Not everybody was individually counted and recorded as they were dumped into the graves. Besides, many death certificates were incorrectly signed off as pneumonia and not influenza.

There was a reason that some people lived, and some people died. It was about where and how they lived, how old they were, where they worked, and who they loved. It was not by chance alone.

Susceptible groups:

Young people under age 29

The previous Influenza epidemic was 1889–90. Those older than 29 had lived through that epidemic and perhaps earlier ones as well, and probably had some degree of acquired immunity. Those 29 and younger were unlikely to have had any exposure to Influenza, and did not have any immunity to it and were among those susceptible.

Four million American men, age range 19 to 31, were inducted into the US Army. Influenza began in the US Army in 1917 and spread throughout the world. The soldiers were young, had no immunity if under 29 years of age, and lived where the epidemic was most active in crowded training camps, on crowded troopships, and at the front.

Pregnant women seemed to be very susceptible to Influenza. In general, pregnant woman were young and, if less than 29 years old, they had no immunity to influenza. The pregnant wives, girlfriends, and fiancées of four million soldiers may have become infected when they visited the troops before the army sailed to Europe. Other women became ill after visiting their influenza-stricken soldiers in hospital.

Immigrants. Minimal information was available in Italian, Yiddish, Russian, etc. Many in the slums lived cheek to jowl in a single poorly ventilated room.[9]

Dock workers had close proximity to sailors and soldiers.

Native Americans. Lengthy ceremonies held around dead bodies helped to spread the infection among the participants. Isolated on distant reservations, Native Americans had little to no modern medical or nursing help. During Covid 19 in 2020, they continued to have high death rates.

Citizens of Philadelphia had special risks. It was a port city, with embarkation points for troops going overseas. It was also a home to naval bases, naval hospitals, shipyards, and close to large military training camps, had large slums, and had many immigrant residents. If that was not enough, they had to deal with incompetent and corrupt city government.

THE OCTOBER 1918 Philadelphia disaster had its origins in the Boston bond rally on September 3. Influenza began to spread throughout all New England. Unfortunately, hundreds of sailors from Boston were then shipped out to the Philadelphia Naval Yard. Within days of their arrival, 600 of them were hospitalized in Philadelphia and Influenza began to spread.

Wilson should have halted troop transfers in the face of an epidemic. The transfer of these Boston sailors to Philadelphia was inexcusable; it was like dousing a burning city with gasoline.

Many shipbuilders, dockworkers, sailors, and soldiers were crowded along the Delaware River waterfront in the twelve shipbuilding yards, and the busy and crowded US naval shipyard. There was significant co-mingling of civilians and military and the disease spread rapidly, starting with the Boston sailors and going from one group to another. A deadly Influenza outbreak was already overwhelming the nearby military base, Camp Dix, 38 miles from Broad Street in Philadelphia.

Philadelphia was run by the corrupt political machine headed by the boss William Vare, who was a Republican congressman. He was a business partner of the mobster Lucky Luciano. Need one say more?

Wilmer Kruson, director of public health, was part of that machine. Despite the objections of most medical experts, he allowed a bond drive parade to proceed, as he was under extreme pressure to meet bond quotas which were considered a gauge of patriotism. The pandemic match was lit on September 28, 1918, as hundreds of thousands of Philadelphians jammed the streets for a parade and bond rally.[10] The incompetence of the corrupt political machine fanned the flames and the pandemic exploded.

Within 72 hours of the parade, every bed in Philadelphia's 31 hospitals was filled and the death rate soared. At the peak of the outbreak, 837 people would die from Influenza on a single October day in 1918 in the City of Brotherly Love, only 140 miles from the White House and Wilson said and did nothing. There would be more than 12,000 deaths from Influenza in Philadelphia, in autumn 1918, making it one of the deadliest places on earth. That compares with 10,000 deaths from Covid in New York City during the six weeks of March–April 2020.[11]

THE US NAVY: The rapid speed of transportation of increasing number of infected troops by train and troop ship only accelerated the whole process. Ocean liners that could cross the Atlantic in ten to twelve days were converted into troop ships. More troops could now be transported faster than ever before. The troops on the move were the vector for influenza, and the US Army was at great risk.

The very crowded conditions on troop ships going back and forth to Europe seemed designed to spread the epidemic. From seaport to seaport, the civilian and navy sailors carried the disease with them, sharing it with their mates in all the ports of the nation and the world. That was how the virus spread from Boston and Freetown and Brest, ports of troop embarkation.

Wilson decided to continue transporting troops despite the opposition of Dr. Gorgas. Wilson would not allow anything to slow down the transfer of US troops to the Western Front. Some US troops arrived at the front with no guns, incomplete uniforms, and having had only two days of infantry training.

The USS Leviathan was a converted passenger ship, that carried large number of troops rapidly across the Atlantic. This was an efficient way for the pandemic to spread. Recall that September 1918 is the peak of the second wave of influenza in the US.

The Leviathan was to sail for Europe Sept. 30, 1918 with 9300 Army troops. Before sailing over 100 men were removed from ship, ill with influenza. Ninety one men died on board the ship, another 300 died a few days after landing at Brest, There were about 1600-2000 cases on board, and thousands more after landing. This was a needless sacrifice of thousands of young men, on just one ship. Men were too delirious to give their name, so these numbers are only estimates. In his zeal to prosecute the war, Wilson was guilty of reckless indifference and dereliction of duty toward his troops.

How can you defend this awful record.? Few of these 9300 troops were ever ready for combat, as the war would be over in one month. The few troops who remained able-bodied spent time arranging hospitalization for their stricken comrades, and organizing burial details. They then needed to reorganize the able-bodied seamen into functional units.

This was a needless sacrifice of thousands of young men, on just one ship. Wilson did not follow the advice of his world class expert, Dr. William Gorgas: stop the troop transports. Didn't Wilson understand Dr. Gorgas when he told him to stop the troop shipments because they were spreading the epidemic worldwide? How can one justify sending sick troops overseas? Was Wilson obsessed with being a war president? On the other hand, the US needed to demonstrate that it was a fighting ally. No pause in the war effort could be tolerated. Keep the pressure on to win the war.

Wilson was apparently more concerned with winning WWI than with controlling the epidemic in the US. This was despite the fact that there were many more civilian deaths than military ones: 675,000 civilian deaths vs 116,000 military deaths, and about half of those deaths were to influenza.

Was Wilson trapped by an inner conflict? We have no record of what he said or felt. The US Army was fighting the largest land battle in US history, the Meuse-Argonne offensive. The Germans were retreating but had not yet surrendered. The US could not stop the troop transport, as we had the Germans are on their last leg . One more push and the war is over. Win the war at all costs. Curtail civil liberties at home, ration food, collect scrap metals. People who died from Influenza were felt to be just another type of war casualty. So, death by Influenza is easily conflated to death in combat.

Postponing a few transport ships would have had little effect on the war, but might have saved thousands of lives, in the US. By October 1918, the Ottoman Empire had surrendered, and both the German and Austrian governments had called for an armistice.

The United States would keep fighting until the very end of the war. "On November 11, 1918, Armistice Day, the American Expeditionary Forces on the Western Front in France suffered more than thirty-five hundred casualties, although it had been known unofficially for two days that the fighting would end that day and known with absolute certainty as of 5 o'clock that morning that it would end at 11 a.m."[13] To continue combat until 11 a.m. was blood lust.

. . .

WHAT WILSON FAILED to do to Combat Influenza: The Pandemic was like a great fire out of control and Wilson was the fire chief who did not respond to the fire alarms. Rome burned while Nero fiddled. Influenza raged and Wilson said and did nothing! Not a little bit. No, he did nothing, zilch, nada. He was grossly negligent and was guilty of dereliction of duty.

Wilson failed to assume personal leadership for the crisis and direct a coordinated national policy. He did not direct the US Public Health Service to provide a plan for fair allocation of resources, especially nurses. He did not follow the advice of his expert, Dr. Gorgas, who had international experience dealing with epidemics. Wilson was an outstanding public speaker, but he did not make any public speeches about the pandemic nor did he make a special address to Congress.

He had wide powers as commander-in-chief to stop recruitment, suspend the draft, quarantine all military bases, stop all military movement by train or ship or truck. At the very least he should have decreased the numbers of troops on board ships and not let any sick soldiers on board. He did none of the above, until the last months of the war.

SEVERAL CIVILIAN FACTORS Helped to Spread the 1918 Epidemic: There was a great shortage of civilian doctors, as about one third of all doctors were in the army. Large numbers of nurses developed influenza because of their close contact with patients, and they were among the first to die. (The toll of health care workers has continued in the COVID era. As of March 2021, 3,700 health care workers had died from Covid 19 during the first year of the pandemic.)

The 1918 public ignored the advice to quarantine the sick and to limit attendance at large public gatherings. They continued to aggregate at huge bond rallies and attended school, theaters, and baseball games.[17]

The United States had a poorly coordinated network of

federal, state, and local public health departments. Informed local leadership frequently was lacking. Several public health commissioners were political hacks. There was haphazard implementation of quarantine rules. Many people thought of the flu as just another aspect of the war, and the dead from Influenza were thought of as just another casualty of war.

Civilians in the port cities, dock workers and their families, sailors on troopships, people living near army camps and near the front lines, railroad workers, health care workers and girlfriends of soldiers were among the first to become ill.

THE US ARMY: The army was deeply involved in the spread of Influenza. US Army training camps in Kansas in 1917 may have been the original site of the epidemic. The increasing mobilization of troops in the US Army created more fuel for the fire. There would be a great number of troops in training camps, on troop ships and trains, and on all the military fronts.

As the soldiers went from training camps to trains, to embarkation ports in US, to troopships, to the docks in England and France, to the front line, and then return to the US, they spread the virus everywhere they went. This was a continuous circle, non-stop, as the war effort continued unabated.

Woodrow Wilson, erstwhile professor of American history, seemed unaware that an American army could easily be destroyed during a pandemic. Over one half of the US Army became infected with influenza during the autumn of 1918, mainly as a direct result of his failure to act. One in every sixty soldiers in the US Army died from Influenza in the autumn of 1918. If this had continued or accelerated, the US Army could have been destroyed. The Armistice occurred just in time.[18]

Why did the Princeton educated Wilson fail to grasp what the unschooled Washington understood 143 years earlier, that an epidemic could destroy the army and needed to be contained as the first war policy?

THE VIRUS: Most important, the virus had mutated to a more lethal strain among the frontline troops in the trenches of Western Europe. In the trenches of Western Front, the massive bombardment and the pervasive choking dust, the tens of thousands of decaying unburied bodies, and the extraordinarily close living conditions, the soaking wet clothes, the man-eating mud, and the gas-warfare-damaged respiratory tracts of the soldiers created a new and toxic environment that favored the mutation of more lethal strains of the virus.

It bears repeating. In the face of this national and worldwide pandemic Woodrow Wilson did absolutely nothing. Fortunately, WWI and the second wave of Influenza epidemic both stopped at about the exact same time during the second week of November 1918.

THE TRUMP RECORD: The 2020 Covid 19 pandemic presented a similar challenge for President Donald Trump. He refused to take ownership of the Covid 19 response. Trump repeated many of Wilson's failures and had some of his own.

In addition, Trump minimized the seriousness of the disease. He injected the issue of xenophobia into the discussion, blaming the Chinese for much of the problem, referring to Covid as China Flu, the Kung Foo Flu, etc. He supported useless and dangerous remedies for Covid, such as bleach and hydroxychloroquine.

He prevented formulation of a national policy for Covid 19, leaving decision making to the states. He left purchase of critical supplies for the states to bid against each other in the open market. He frequently did not wear a mask in public and made fun of those that did. He silenced scientists who disagreed with him. He withdrew the US from the World Health Organization, disregarding the critical need for international cooperation during a pandemic. He continued or did not discourage large outdoor and indoor political rallies which were super spreader events such as the Sturgis, South Dakota motorcycle rally, his Tulsa political rally, and his White House lawn reception for Justice Amy Coney Barrett. His performance was similar to Wilson's, and so the disaster of 1918 was needlessly repeated in 2020.

Contrast that record with the following: In the summer of 2005, President George W. Bush began reading *"The Great Influenza"* by John Barry. He couldn't put it down. When he returned to Washington, he called Fran Townsend, his top homeland security adviser, into the Oval Office and told her to create a national strategy for dealing with pandemics.[14] Thus was born the nation's most comprehensive pandemic plan, a playbook that included diagrams for a global early warning system, funding to develop new, rapid vaccine technology, and a robust national stockpile of critical supplies, such as face masks and ventilators. The plan would be sustained by an office in the White House.[15]

The effort was intense over the ensuing three years of Bush's presidency, including exercises where cabinet officials gamed out their responses to disastrous biological scenarios. Much of the plan, but not all of it, continued under President Barack Obama. Displaying a lack of foresight, the Trump administration closed the planning office, abandoned the plans, and dispersed the staff.[16] The result was unmitigated disaster when Covid 19 appeared in 2020. There was no plan, no office, and no trained staff in place to implement a response.

Fortunately, President Trump was able to jump start the world-wide vaccine production program. He has to receive great credit for that accomplishment.

. . .

BOOKS AND PAINTINGS about the epidemic: [20] These include *Look Homeward Angel*, a 1929 novel by Thomas Wolfe and *Pale Horse Pale Rider*, Katherine Anne Porter's 1939 war novella. Paintings include *The Interior of a Hospital Tent*, 1918, painted by John Singer Sargent, and *Self Portrait with the Spanish flu*, 1919, by Edward Munch.

14

DISASTER IN PARIS 1919, STALEMATE IN THE US SENATE

Following Cleveland's boat ride up the East River, the next presidential coverup occurred during the administration of Woodrow Wilson. The outcome was disaster for the nation and the world.

Woodrow Wilson was unique in our parade of presidents. He had very good care by an excellent physician who participated in and personally benefitted from the massive cover-up that took place.

On May 28, 1906, Wilson suddenly lost vision in his left eye, probably due to a *retinal hemorrhage*.[1] This may have been a harbinger for his 1918 stroke, but that remains a controversial medical topic.

Wilson appeared to be in good health when he was elected president in 1912. During a 1913 inaugural luncheon, Wilson's sister fell and cut her forehead. Dr. Cary Grayson, a Navy physician was on the spot and neatly sutured her wound.[2] Wilson was so impressed that he offered Grayson the post of White House physician. Dr. Grayson was a competent, well-trained physician who lived at the White House until his own marriage, and became very close to the Wilson family.

He was best man at the wedding of one of the Wilson daughters.

He was promoted several grades, jumping ahead of dozens of naval officers in rank. In 1913, he was a lieutenant; by 1916, he was promoted to rear admiral.

"He sutured up the sister so carefully that now he is an admiral in the US Navy." Apologies to Gilbert and Sullivan, (HMS Pinafore) words by ELG, music by Arthur Sullivan.

Grayson provided some of the medical care to the first Mrs. Wilson who died of renal failure in 1914. After her death Grayson introduced Wilson to his friend, Edith Bolling Galt, a Washington, DC socialite. She was related to both Pocahontas and Thomas Jefferson and in 1915, she became the second Mrs. Wilson.

President Wilson and Dr. Grayson felt indebted to each other. This was complemented by the already close friendship of Mrs. Wilson and Dr. Grayson. So, the bonds between Woodrow and Edith Wilson and Cary Grayson were intense, intimate, and multi-layered, and Grayson responded with complete loyalty to the Wilsons. Most physicians are reluctant to be in such intimate extra-professional relations with their patients, as the potential for conflict of interest is high.

Wilson was re-elected by a narrow margin in 1916, claiming to have kept America out of the war. But after Germany resumed unrestricted submarine warfare on February 1, 1917, the US declared war on Germany on April 6, 1917. That state of war concluded with the Armistice November 1918, and Wilson went to Paris twice to negotiate a peace treaty.

During his second Paris trip, in April 1919, Wilson developed an illness with fever and a cough that was probably Influenza.[3] What is the evidence for that? The third wave of the Influenza epidemic had just occurred in the spring of 1919 and Paris was involved with thousands of cases. Wilson was in the correct time and place to be infected by the third wave. A member of Wilson's staff became ill with Influenza at the same time, and the young man went on to die. Dr. Grayson, who was in Paris with Wilson at that time, made the president's diagnosis of Influenza based upon his first-hand observation. Grayson was a competent physician who had spent a year training with William Osler at Johns Hopkins. For all these reasons, Grayson's evaluation is presumed to be correct.

Following this febrile illness, Wilson had a marked change in personality which persisted for the rest of his life. No one can say with certainty what was the cause of these mental changes. Was this a *post-viral encephalopathy*, or was this a small stroke? No matter the cause, following his Influenza he began to exhibit strange persona behavior

This becomes the most important medical episode in modern history. No other medical illness ever had such an impact upon the historical events that were forthcoming.[4] The world awaited his trip to Paris with such high hopes. His portrait was everywhere. Flowers, parades, and huge crowds greeted Wilson everywhere he went. But his brain disease cut him down to size, and he accomplished very little.

What poetic justice that the man who helped spread the epidemic, was himself infected in 1919, and lost his mind as a result. Herbert Hoover, who was part of the US delegation at Versailles, said Wilson's mind had lost its resiliency and he no longer had a grasp of the issues.[5] The consequences of these mental changes were enormous, and tragic. At the conference in Paris, Wilson no longer had the intellect and the mental toughness required to oppose the punitive demands of Italy and France that were so resented by Germany and probably helped spark WWII. The European diplomats played him like a fiddle, and the world was not made safe for democracy.

Nor did Wilson have the ability to secure passage of his own plan. Only one of his Fourteen Points made it into the final treaty; the one that established The League of Nations. The others were excised (freedom of the seas, prohibition of secret treaties, reduction in armaments, free trade).

France and Belgium got their revenge with a vengeance, exemplified by the food blockade resulting in famine in Germany and 500,000 deaths. Germany had signed the 1918 Armistice with the understanding that Wilson's Fourteen Points would be enforced. The Allies reneged on that. It was fashionable to criticize Wilson's Fourteen Points, noting that there were only Ten Commandments. The Allies kept all their secret treaties, control of the ocean, colonies, and exclusive economic systems. They occupied the Rhineland with French troops from Africa. The dragon's teeth that they planted in 1919 sprang up in 1933 as Hitler and the Nazis.[6]

Back to reality. Wilson's loss of intellect in 1919 at the Paris Peace Conference was an unmitigated disaster. There would be no world peace, and the world was not made safe for democracy.[7] The carnage of World War I had been in vain and would be renewed in 1939. This was the greatest impact made on history by the health of a U.S. president.

Upon returning to Washington, Wilson's strange behavior continued. He was inflexible, became obsessed with trivia, and began to have paranoid thoughts. He personally tried to apprehend speeding automobile drivers. He also threatened to break off relations with England, taking offense over a risqué joke told by a British diplomat. Wilson was now intellectually damaged.

The League of Nations was still alive and on his return to Washington, Wilson engaged the US Senate in discussions about US entry into the League. That too failed. The following is an account of that failure.

The 1918 elections gave control of the US Senate to the Republicans with a 49–47 majority. Recall that in 1918 there were 96 senators and that the Constitution required a two-thirds vote (64 votes) to ratify a treaty. Since 46 of the 47 Democrats supported the treaty, the Democrat Wilson needed at least 18 Republican votes to reach the 64-vote threshold.

This 64-vote total was within reach as there were probably

31 Republican senators who would have voted for a treaty with some modifications.

Note the treaty clause of the Constitution. "The President shall have Power by and with the Advice and Consent of the Senate, to make Treaties, provided two-thirds of the Senators present concur."

So, if only 90 senators showed up for the vote, only 60 votes would be needed. And it is in this volatile world of changing quorums, etc., treaties fail or succeed. Complex Senate rules about abstaining and paired voting only add to the difficulty of managing a treaty through the Senate. So, it will need a continuous, hands-on political effort to create a two-thirds vote required to pass a treaty.

Obviously, Wilson needed to negotiate with the Republicans to pass the treaty. The Republicans offered several modifications to the peace treaty. Even though the French and British notified Wilson that the Republican modifications were acceptable to them, Wilson refused to negotiate. He was inflexible and must share the blame for the failure of the US to ratify the peace treaty. Defeat at Paris; defeat at the US Senate.

After Wilson's plan was rejected in the Senate, he began a nationwide trip in August 1919 to win public support for the unmodified peace treaty. Almost all of Wilson's medical records are missing, so all the following is a likely re-creation based on incomplete information.

On September 25, 1919, while boarding a train in Pueblo, Colorado, Wilson showed slurred speech, unsteady gait, and left-sided facial weakness. That was probably an episode of *transient cerebral ischemia*. The brain cells are injured but not killed and symptoms last a from a few minutes to a few hours. The Wilsons returned immediately to Washington, DC, 1,651 miles by rail. Upon return to Washington, Wilson was greatly improved.

But that changed on the morning of October 2, 1919 in the White House. Wilson then suffered complete left-sided paralysis and was no longer *compos mentis*. It was apparent that Wilson was disabled with a major *stroke*; there is no question about this. A stroke implies that the brain cells are destroyed and symptoms are permanent. Over a varying period of time, patients may have some recovery, but that involves a complex process that I will not go into.

Wilson was physically and mentally unable to discharge the "Powers and Duties of the said Office" of the presidency. He was paralyzed and could not speak clearly. He could not reason. He was confused and very weak. He hardly ate and was confined to bed for almost two months. His disability changed the history of the world, and not in a good way.

Once again let's look at the US Constitution, Article II, Section 1:

"In Case of the Removal of the President from Office, or of his Death, Resignation, or Inability to discharge the Powers and Duties of the said Office, the Same shall devolve on the Vice President."

According to the Constitution, it appeared that the powers and duties had automatically devolved onto Vice President Thomas Marshall, and he should have become the president.[8]

Vice President Thomas Marshall was a capable politician, especially in the Senate where he had successfully managed several controversial wartime measures. He was also a strong proponent of the League of Nations and, given the opportunity, might have successfully provided the leadership needed for ratification of the peace treaty. But Wilson was not willing to vacate the presidency.

Marshall never seized the day to proclaim that he was president. Why did Marshall shirk his responsibility? Was it dereliction of duty, or loyalty to Wilson? He refused to unilaterally assume the presidency and was waiting for a Congressional resolution of support which never materialized. That certificate of Wilson's disability was never written. Who was supposed to write it? Again, there was no constitutional requirement for such a disability certificate, nor for any Congressional resolution. Nevertheless, according to the Constitution, Marshall was president since Wilson clearly had an *"Inability to discharge the Powers and Duties of the said Office"* of the presidency.

Absent a joint Congressional resolution declaring the president to be incapacitated, Marshall refused to unilaterally assume the presidency. That supporting Congressional resolution had significant support, but it was blocked by anti-treaty senators. They reasoned that the capable Marshall might indeed have the political skills necessary to ratify the peace treaty. They preferred a disabled President Wilson and an unratified treaty to a capable President Marshall and a ratified treaty. The resolution never passed, and Marshall never announced or proclaimed that he was president. All the many Democratic and Republican Congressional leaders and Democratic cabinet members had taken an oath to defend and protect the Constitution. They all shirked their duty.

This was an historic failure of the Constitution to provide a process to put Marshall in the Oval Office. This turned out to be a disaster for the world. If only VP Marshall had the courage of John Tyler to seize the power that was available to him.

Thomas Marshall refused to unilaterally take office. The cabinet had been kept out of the loop. The Congress was engrossed in the usual party politics, especially revolving around ratification of the peace treaty, and the courts were silent. The president was missing in action and only Secretary of State Robert Lansing seemed to care.

After Wilson's completed stroke, when the paralysis became permanent, there were several opportunities to reveal his disability, but Grayson the doctor now became Grayson the kingmaker. Never before nor since has any physician wielded so much political power.

Several days after the return to Washington from Colorado, Secretary of State Lansing met Dr. Grayson and Wilson's private secretary, Joseph Tumulty. Lansing quoted the Constitution's Article II, Section 1 devolvement of powers clause and advocated that VP Marshall replace the disabled Wilson as president. Dr. Grayson responded that he would never certify Wilson's disability and that ended that threat.

A cabinet meeting was held a few days later without the president in attendance. Dr. Grayson delivered a message from the president asking by whose authority the cabinet was meeting? Grayson said nothing about Wilson's stroke and only spoke in general terms. The cabinet backed down and said nothing more of significance. Lansing had scheduled the meeting, and that fiasco ended any influence he had in government. Since he was still in office with no instructions or influence, US foreign policy came to a halt. Foreign diplomats were not being accredited to the US and foreign policy was stagnant After several months in limbo, Lansing finally resigned in February 1920. He was replaced by Frank Polk and then Bainbridge Colby.

Wilson was totally disabled and remained so for at least the first five months following his stroke. For the first two months, he barely got out of bed, spoke only a few words, slept for much of the time, and was incapable of any meaningful decision making. Apart from his wife, Edith Wilson, Dr. Grayson, and his butler, Ike Hoover, he had no visitors. Over the next few months, he made very slow progress.

After a few months he got out of bed and received a few visitors. Yet he remained incapable of performing even the most menial of tasks, let alone fulfill his executive duties. What a dilemma. Woodrow Wilson was disabled and unable to perform as president.

The president of the United States had not been seen for months; was he dead or alive? In December 1919, after President Wilson had some neurological improvement, Mrs. Wilson arranged a tableau for a select group of senators. The president sat on a chaise lounge with his non-paralyzed right side facing the audience of senators. He had grown a beard to mask his facial paralysis.

One of the senators said, "We are praying for you, Mr. President."[9] Wilson tersely replied, "Which way?"

～

THAT WAS the extent of congressional oversight. It is difficult to explain why the world seemed to acquiesce in this farce that everything was alright. Only the theater of the absurd comes close to interpreting this.

The United States did not appear to have a foreign policy. Only a few medical bulletins noted that the president was alive but tired. Political vacancies piled up, laws and other documents were not signed.

"No worries, everything is OK, or nothing was OK." Who was in charge? Better still, was anyone in charge?[10] Power abhors a vacuum and into the breech stepped Edith Wilson, assisted by Dr. Grayson and Joseph Tumulty. She performed many functions for the president, but she insisted that the president made all the decisions. Mrs. Wilson disliked Marshall and so he was removed from any participation in the government. She gathered reports, received legislation, etc. Bills were signed by Mrs. Wilson or by the president, and no one knows how that was possible. Did Mrs. Wilson forge her husband's signature? Did she hold the pen while he made a few scratches at the bottom of a letter? Some documents were rubber stamped with the presidential signature. She pretended that the president was in charge, when in fact she was. Mrs. Wilson set the agenda, screened all visitors, and few made it into Wilson's bedroom where he lay bed-ridden.

Dr. Grayson, along with Mrs. Wilson, was part of the inner circle that prevented people from seeing the sick president. Tumulty became the spokesman to the outside world. So, unelected citizens responsible to no one effectively took over control of the government. The authors of Section 4 of the 25th Amendment may have had Edith Wilson in mind when they wrote about the involuntary removal of a disabled president.

What happened was an historic cover-up that led to the usurpation of the presidency by his wife, his physician, and his private secretary Joseph Tumulty, none of whom is mentioned in the devolve clause or anywhere else in the Constitution. In effect, this troika overthrew the presidency of the US. Edith Wilson, Carey Grayson, and Joseph Tumulty had assumed the presidency, which had devolved unto them.[11]

As long as the cover-up remained in place, and Wilson remained alive, Marshall would never become president. Tragically for the world, that meant a Treaty of Paris would never pass the US Senate, and the US never entered the League of Nations.

What Mrs. Wilson could not do was to fight for the Treaty.[12] That required a personal approach by the president utilizing all his political skills, prestige, and charisma. As Wilson's health had significantly declined, the chances of ratification of the treaty were minimal.

This became an historical failure of the Constitution to provide an orderly process of succession, to install Marshall as president, and to remove Wilson from office. The peaceful constitutional transition of power had failed.

The most important presidential task of the moment was to provide leadership in promoting and fighting for the peace treaty.[13] Wilson was physically unable to do that, and Marshall never had the chance. What an unmitigated disaster. No illness had ever caused so much harm.

The great newspapers *New York Times* and *Washington Post* failed to comment on Wilson's absence from the public, and were very slow and incomplete in their news accounts.

Foreign diplomats never saw the president. Why were the foreign nations silent? Why didn't someone go to the federal courts? Was this a wide conspiracy or just a cockamamie scheme of a loving wife, who overreached a bit?

Why did the cabinet accept Wilson's paralysis and dementia? What happened to congressional oversight or even impeachment? But the Republicans who controlled the senate were not unhappy with Wilson's disability. Absent Wilson's leadership, they figured correctly that the peace treaty would not be ratified. This act by the Republicans had them place party above country, and this was the party of Lincoln.

Yet in fairness to the Republicans, in 1920 they put forward a good faith plan to adopt the treaty with reservations. There was still hope for the US to enter the League. The result of direct US involvement would have led to some change in history. Who knows? Could it have been worse than World War II?

At the end of the day, the treaty was still alive in the Senate. There were only 84 Senators present and voting. That meant that only 56 votes were required to ratify the treaty.

The Republicans voted 28–12 to support the treaty. This plan had the votes for ratification until Wilson intervened and persuaded some Democrats to vote no. The Democratic vote was 21–23 to oppose the treaty. The final vote on March 19, 1920, was 49 to 35 to ratify the treaty so the vote fell only seven votes short of ratification.

Wilson had helped to kill his own child, the peace treaty and its infant, the League of Nations. Why would he do that? Wilson didn't cause World War II, but look at the opportunity that he had to make an enduring peace. So close. Imagine no war.

IMAGINE FOR A MOMENT ANOTHER WORLD, with a different outcome. Wilson does not become ill in Paris. His intellect is intact and he manages to have most of his Fourteen Points adopted. The food blockade is ended, punitive measures are few and far between. The Allies agree to support democracy in

Germany. Wilson does not oppose racial equality among the nations and Japan signs the peace treaty, secret trade pacts are abolished.

When he returns to the US, he compromises with the Republicans with the least reservations. And voila! The US enters the League of Nations. Imagine no World War II, no Hitler, no atomic bomb. Sixty million people are not killed in combat, death camps or in aerial bombardments, or famine or typhus. Can you imagine that? Wasn't Wilson supposed to be history's man of destiny? This could have happened.

Oh sure, wishful thinking. Get real. Yet only twenty-six years later in 1945, FDR picked up Wilson's fallen torch and led the western world to victory and peace. The United Nations has been in business since April 1945. Excepting the civil war in the former Yugoslavia, Europe was free from war for seventy-seven years. Sadly, the Russian invasion of Ukraine in 2022 ended FDR's dream of peace in Europe.

Back to reality. Wilson's loss of intellect in 1919 at the Paris Peace Conference was an unmitigated disaster. Wilson's encephalopathy paved the way for World War II. This was the greatest impact made on history by the health of a U.S. president.

What makes it worse was that the Wilsons were usurpers and unfit to be in power. Thomas Marshall was the legal president or else the Constitution is meaningless. Finally, with the election of Warren Harding in 1920, the transitional process eventually returned to a legal constitutional basis.

The loyalty that began with a sutured forehead, held up despite enormous pressure. Dr. Grayson issued a bulletin that only stated that the president was a very sick man. Dr. Francis Dercum, the chief consultant to the president, ordered that all bad news and visitors be kept from the president.

No diagnosis was ever mentioned to the public, congress or to Vice President Marshall. Grayson never made any public statement that Wilson had suffered a stroke, and again most significantly, the presidency never devolved upon Vice President Marshall.

About five months into his stroke, Wilson began to make some improvement. He got out of bed and learned to walk with a cane. He ate regular meals and regained his lost weight. He began to meet people and went outside for automobile trips to the country side. He began to speak more fluently, but his sharp intellect was gone. He probably was no longer completely disabled, but still not fit for office. He was only a shadow of his former self. For the remainder of his presidency, he made modest but slow improvement.

Wilson did not attend a cabinet meeting until April 1920, almost six months after his stroke. Although he had made a partial recovery, his feeble condition shocked cabinet members. Most of Wilson's cabinet still did not know the true state of his health. This meeting was called by Wilson, who spoke in a weak voice and told a few jokes, followed by moments of silence. Mrs. Wilson mercifully ending the meeting after about one hour. There would be no further opportunities to confront Wilson about his fitness to serve.

The press began to publish stories about Wilson's stroke, sometimes in a positive way; i.e. "the president continues to make improvement." But by and large, the public was kept in the dark. So much for democracy. By February of 1920, news of the president's stroke began to be reported in the press. However, the full details of Woodrow Wilson's disability and his wife's management of his affairs were not revealed to the American public at the time.

There was also a domestic crisis during Wilson's incapacity. Race riots occurred throughout the US. Black soldiers still on active duty and in uniform were being lynched, and received no protection from the federal government. There were no plans to address high inflation, collapse of farm prices, high unemployment, and continuing industrial unrest and strikes.

There was a continuing attack on civil liberties. Prosecutions for anti-war activity continued under the Sedition Act of 1918 even though the war was over. The Red Raids began, and US residents were being deported to the USSR. Woodrow Wilson had no knowledge of these raids that took place without his authorization. They were led by Attorney General Mitchell Palmer and his assistant John Hoover, before he became J. Edgar Hoover. During Wilson's lengthy disability, Hoover and Mitchell suppressed civil liberties, their only restraint being Assistant Secretary of Labor Louis Post, an unsung hero.

Wilson received competent medical care as far as we know, but he was disabled and unable to perform as president. Do you know of any similar political disaster in American history?

For the remainder of her life, Edith Wilson insisted that her husband performed all his presidential duties after his stroke. There is no evidence to support that. Recently, Dr. Grayson's family released his private papers. These do not support Mrs. Wilson's views about the president's ability to discharge the powers and duties of the office.

Let's return to Wilson's high ratings in the presidential polls. Wilson usually makes the top ten, and the esteemed historian Arthur Schlesinger, Jr. ranked him as number six. How did they arrive at that conclusion? Surely, his flagrant racism and his dereliction of duty during the 1918 Influenza drags his ranking toward the bottom.

After he died in 1924, Wilson left behind three devoted daughters, a loving wife, and a loyal son in-law, all of whom protected and promoted his legacy. Mrs. Wilson remained a Democratic Party insider for many years, including chair of the women's division.

Her son-in-law, William McAdoo, ran for the Democratic nomination for president in 1920 and 1924, and was elected an US senator from California in 1932. In 1933, Wilson's protégé, FDR, became the 33rd US president. Mrs. Wilson accompanied FDR to Congress on December 8, 1941, for the Day of

Infamy speech, and was JFK's guest at his inauguration in 1961.

The following organizations were established and dedicated to advancing the aims and memory of Woodrow Wilson.

- *Woodrow Wilson School of Public and International Affairs at Princeton*
- *Woodrow Wilson International Center for Scholars, in Washington, D.C.*, established as part of the Smithsonian Institution by an act of Congress in 1968. It is a highly recognized think tank, ranked among the top ten in the world.
- *Woodrow Wilson Foundation* founded in 1945 has awarded fellowships to more than 22,000 scholars, who now include 15 Nobel Laureates, 38 MacArthur "Genius Grant" Fellows, and 19 Pulitzer Prize winners. In 1921 FDR would serve as chairman of the foundation's national committee.

What an incredible group of politically connected and talented academic people who must have some allegiance to the legacy of Woodrow Wilson. Wilson may have maintained his reputation through the support of well-placed politicians and thousands of scholars indebted to one of his programs.

Wilson made a futile gesture to run for a third term, but that never got off the ground. Instead, the Democratic ticket in 1920 was Governor Cox of Ohio with FDR as VP candidate. They were crushed in a landslide by the Republican ticket of Warren Harding and Calvin Coolidge. In March 1921, Warren Harding was inaugurated, and there were no issues about the legitimacy of the election. The baton had been picked up by Harding. Mercifully, the Edith Wilson presidency had come to an end.

15

FRANKLIN DELANO ROOSEVELT

It is appropriate to segue directly from Woodrow Wilson to FDR, as there were many connections and similarities between them. Their most direct connection was that FDR served as President Wilson's assistant secretary of navy.

William Bullet and Breckinridge Long served as diplomats for both Wilson and FDR. Josephus Daniels was a confidant of both Wilson and FDR, serving as secretary of the navy for Wilson and thirteen years later as ambassador to Mexico for FDR. Daniel's son, Johnathan, was FDR's press secretary in 1945.

Wilson and FDR both focused upon post-war international organizations as a way of keeping world peace; for Wilson the League of Nations and for FDR, the United Nations. Both men were involved in medical cover-ups that featured missing medical records. Cary Grayson served as a medical advisor for both men. Both men's medical cover-ups led to diplomatic failure at Paris 1919 and then at Yalta 1945. Both men were influenza victims in 1919, and both suffered severe adverse effects. Both men were stroke victims. Wilson lost his mind and FDR lost his life.

As part of his military duties, FDR toured the Western Front in 1918. In October 1918, he returned home aboard the infamous troopship USS *Leviathan*, along with thousands of troops. There was an outbreak of influenza on board, and FDR became one of many who were infected. Unfortunately for FDR, his illness evolved into bilateral pneumonia. He was desperately ill and taken off the ship by ambulance, but was treated at home and recovered. While he was home in bed, Eleanor Roosevelt discovered his love letters to Lucy Mercer which FDR had carried with him to and from Europe. This discovery destroyed his intimate relationship with Eleanor, although they remained married.

15 A. Polio and Paralysis and Liberation

Polio is usually an acute childhood disease caused by the polio virus. It is very contagious and is spread by the fecal/oral route. There are episodic epidemics, as well as sporadic cases. Most cases have minimal to no symptoms, and so most parents are unaware that their child has polio. Less than 5 percent of polio cases are paralytic. Only about one percent of all cases result in permanent paralysis, and fatality is uncommon.[1]

The virus spreads from person to person via infected water or food. Summertime activities puts children close together at the beach, summer camp, playing together and sharing together from sandbox to sandlots. Most children contract polio by playing with other children during the summer, late August being the peak time.

But FDR was not most children and spent most of his time alone, schooled at home, and sequestered from other children. So, he did not have much opportunity to contract polio as a child.[2]

In August 1921, the 39-year-old FDR attended a Boy Scout

Jamboree and helped to extinguish a forest fire. Most observers believe that the Jamboree and the close contact with the Boy Scouts was the source of the polio virus that paralyzed him several days later at Campobello Island. In 1921, there was no vaccine and no antiviral treatment, but FDR began a long and fruitless search for a cure. He continuously worked on his physical therapy. As FDR got polio as an adult, it is not surprising that he did not have the classic signs and symptoms of childhood polio. A good argument has been made that FDR was paralyzed by *Guillain-Barré syndrome* and not polio. They both may lead to varying degrees of paralysis. This argument is best left to expert neurologists.

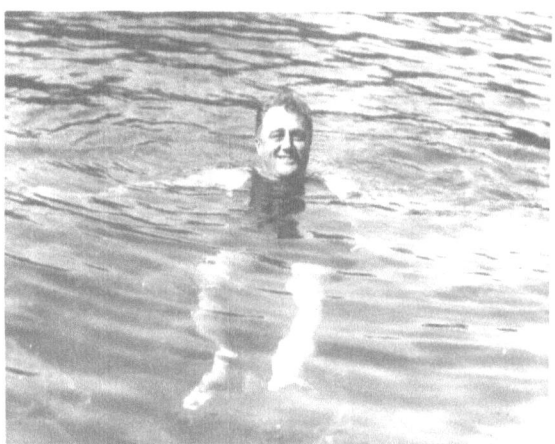

Image 13: FDR swimming in the pool at Warm Springs, 1920s

During his long fruitless search for a cure, FDR came upon the semi-abandoned spa located in Warm Springs, Georgia. Water came from the ground at a constant 88 degrees F, and was said to have therapeutic value. Using two-thirds of his personal fortune, FDR purchased and restored the spa to become the only polio hospital in the US. No one was cured there, but lives were restored, self-esteem regenerated, and enthusiasm reigned.

During the 1920s, Roosevelt underwent a metamorphosis at Warm Springs from Franklin Roosevelt, the aristocratic lightweight dilettante, to FDR, the great humanitarian and world leader. Swimming in the warm waters of the pool with paralyzed children had anointed him with a powerful sense of hope that great things were possible for the children, himself, and the nation.

Politically, this came to life as the New Deal and its myriad of programs. For FDR the politician, the pools of Warm Springs inspired him to think that great things could be accomplished,

The Ford Motor Co. built FDR a special hand-controlled automobile that he drove thousands of miles around the countryside of Meriwether County, Georgia where Warm Springs is located. He was liberated from the world of the wheelchair to hold hundreds of one-on-one encounters with local residents and learned first-hand of the hardships of rural life.[3] The back roads of Meriwether County became the the post-graduate school of the political education of FDR. He specialized in empathy, spontaneous public speaking, and pressing the flesh. In the 1932 presidential election, he won 98 percent of the vote in Meriwether County.

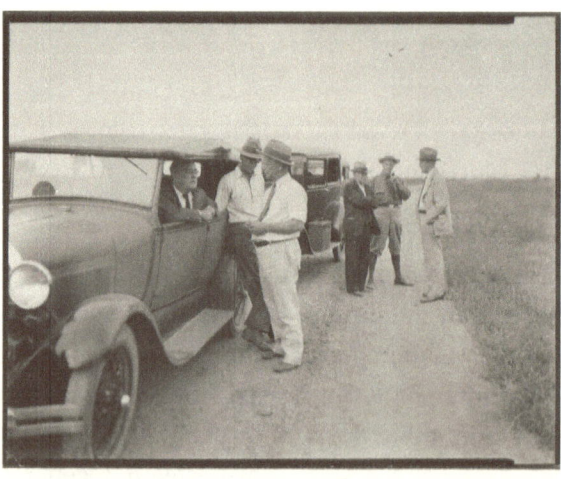

Image 14: FDR Greeting the voters of Georgia, 1920s

From the mid-1920s onward, FDR led a full and active life. He went swimming and sailing; rode horses; canoed; went fishing; drove his own car; and traveled widely. He had a law practice with Basil O'Connor, and together they created and ran the Warm Springs Foundation, which morphed into the March of Dimes. He was fluent in French and when he had lunch with Albert Einstein they conversed in German.

Among his other roles, FDR was president of Greater NY Council of Boy Scouts and a member of the Harvard Board of Overseers. A lifelong Democrat, he was elected governor of New York for two terms and president of the US for four terms. He was a major Allied strategist for World War II for both the Atlantic and Pacific theaters. He planned and supervised building the atomic bomb, and he made it US policy to drop the atomic bomb to win the war.

FDR traveled thousands of miles worldwide in the war effort and met with Stalin and Churchill and many other world leaders. He had many friends and carried on intimate affairs with several women over a period of twenty-four years, none of whom were named Eleanor.

FDR was not disabled by polio for any constitutional purposes. He was able to meet the constitutional requirements *"to be able to discharge the powers and of the said office"* president.

He was hardly a disabled man. Despite his paralysis, FDR was a healthy vigorous man, but his paralysis was always hidden. He could not walk unassisted, but the public never saw that. He rarely was seen in public in a wheelchair. Learning to disguise his paralysis made FDR an expert in duplicity and legerdemain. One way to give the illusion that he was in motion was the frequent photographs and occasional movies of him sailing, swimming, and driving his car, especially with the top down. By holding on to one of his sons, he could ambulate a few steps, usually to a public podium, which gave the illusion that he was walking.[4] He also wore leg braces to support his moving about.

His grandson, Curtis Roosevelt, commented upon FDR's "sense of hope, his creativity, love of a good time, having fun." Other commentators noted the power of FDR's personality, his charisma, and public speaking skills.[5]

Note all the medical metaphors used by FDR in his speeches:[6]

The US was a paralyzed nation (1933); War was seen as a contagion (1937); Need to "quarantine" the aggressors (1937); Doctor New Deal replaced by Doctor Win the War (1943).

15B. FDR's Contributions to Medical Care

FDR was the first president publicly identified and involved with a medical illness: polio.

There had been a long and inglorious history of shaming patients who had infectious diseases. From leprosy in the Bible to AIDS of modern times, infectious disease has been viewed as something dirty. Accordingly, the patients were also seen as unclean and even immoral. Children with polio paralysis bore the additional stigma of being in a wheelchair or on crutches and were hidden from view and isolated. FDR helped change those attitudes with his leadership.[7] He became a facilitator and a promoter of physical rehabilitation that repaired the broken spirit of the polio patients and removed the shame and ostracism of having a paralyzing infectious disease.

At Warm Springs, FDR had been a patient, a fundraiser, a philanthropist, an inventor of medical devices, and a health care provider. He restored and upgraded Warm Springs spa with his inheritance and created a first-class modern center for treating polio. He promoted the use of hydrotherapy as a useful tool along the path to recovery. He invented a new type of crutch useful for polio patients and invented a device to measure muscle strength. Though their paralysis made only minimal improvement, the children learned the skills that enabled them to cope. Their lives would change dramatically. Hope was restored. They would go from a sense of shame to one of acceptance and participation; from the exile of the back room, to full participation in society. The children went swimming, graduated from school, got married, had their own children, taught school, became concert violinists and lawyers, and led the fight for physical access for all Americans.

Along with law partner Basil O 'Connor, he was a great benefactor of research, and created the March of Dimes which over the years has raised hundreds of millions of dollars in the fight against polio and other childhood diseases. Jonas Salk and Albert Sabin both were recipients of March of Dimes funds which helped financed their research and discovery of their respective polio vaccines.

15 C. Hypertension, Congestive Heart Failure, and Yalta

With the onset of FDR's heart failure in the winter of 1943–44, we will obtain the trifecta of a disabled president, an incompetent physician, and massive worldwide cover-up.

Dr. Cary Grayson had a second act after Wilson, serving as a medical advisor to FDR. When FDR was inaugurated as president in 1933, he asked his friend Grayson for a recommendation for the position of White House physician. Since most of FDR's prior ailments had been upper respiratory infections such as tonsillitis and sinusitis, Grayson recommended Dr Ross McIntire, a career US Navy ENT (Ear, Nose and Throat) doctor to be the president's physician. He could take care of FDR's many ENT problems, and he had a reputation for being discrete. Grayson was an expert in this area, as we have seen.

The appointment seemed appropriate, and Dr. McIntire became White House physician, and was also appointed surgeon general of the navy. McIntire's dual appointment as surgeon general of the Navy and White House physician was unique. This was the first time both positions were filled by the same person.

The White House physician was usually a serving US Navy medical officer. There have also been civilians and US Army officers serving in the position.

As a result of his dual appointments, McIntire was promoted to Admiral. By all accounts McIntire was a good wartime navy surgeon general, commanding 169,000 men and women. One statistic says it all. During World War II, about 98 percent of wounded marines and sailors survived their wounds.

However, his performance as White House physician was troubling. It was probably one job too many. As White House physician McIntire became a member of FDR's entourage and saw him every day. His daily exam of FDR consisted of a brief early morning bedside visit, where he would also check FDRs pulse.

That was it, a perfunctory examination at best. McIntire would also administer a dose of nose drops and sinus sprays, usually *vaso-constrictors* that may have played a role in FDR's well-documented onset of hypertension in 1937. The drops and spray containing vaso-constrictors often raised one's blood pressure.[9]

The consequences of FDR's high blood pressure were the following: onset of heart failure in 1944 and sudden death from cerebral hemorrhage in April 1945. Available treatment of hypertension in 1937 would have consisted of staying on a low salt diet, taking sedatives, getting a lot of rest, and stopping the nose drops and sinus sprays. There is no evidence that any of these were done.

In December 1943, FDR returned from Tehran Conference with a chronic cough and fatigue. For the next three months, he spent almost the entire day in bed. His functional capacity was greatly decreased, but the Constitution did not provide a remedy short of resignation. That would not happen as FDR was committed to remain in office until the end of the war.

The heroes of the story then became FDR's daughter, Anna Roosevelt, and Dr. Howard Bruenn, who did the right things for the right reasons.[10] Dr. McIntire had said that FDR's symptoms were due to the flu, but Anna Roosevelt was not satisfied with that explanation. She noted that after many weeks her father was not getting any better. She insisted upon obtaining a second medical opinion and she prevailed. Her advocacy was not surprising, as she had moved into the White House and had become the White House hostess. Anna had also become one of FDRs personal assistants, since Missy LeHand was then out of commission. Missy LeHand had been the indispensable companion, private secretary, and chief of staff. In 1941, she suffered a serious stroke that left her disabled. She continued to live in the White house, and FDR changed his will and left her two thirds of his estate. But she pre-deceased FDR in 1944.

Anna had big shoes to fill and few people appreciated how well she performed. When Anna was chosen to accompany FDR to Yalta in 1945, the importance of her status became apparent for all to see.

In March of 1944, McIntire arranged for FDR to be examined by a 40-year-old US Navy physician, Dr. Howard Bruenn, who had been an academic cardiologist at Columbia University prior to his enlistment. McIntire had made an excellent choice. He had answered Anna's concerns about her father's health. Since he was Bruenn's commanding officer, McIntire could keep close tabs on the situation and control any issues that might evolve.

Upon examination, Bruenn found FDR to be in severe congestive heart failure, a diagnosis supported by EKG and chest X-ray findings. FDR also had marked hypertension, and he was cyanotic (blue) about his fingers. How did McIntire miss such obvious findings?[11]

Most of FDR's clinical records are missing, so there is no objective way to judge McIntire. Perhaps McIntire left it to other doctors to make the tough calls, leaving McIntire to be an administrator or maybe a facilitator. With so many critical administrative responsibilities, McIntire's clinical skills might have atrophied from disuse. The familiarity of the daily routine may have left him unprepared to appreciate what was going on right in front of him.

Directing a huge worldwide medical organization during World War II was a full-time job. How can you do that and also be a good clinician? It probably is not possible. McIntire may have been an excellent ENT doctor, and he may have been an excellent surgeon general, but he was not excellent in internal medicine. His mistake had been to wait too long before obtaining a cardiac consultation for FDR who had been bedridden for weeks. The situation was clearly beyond his competence, and he should have recognized that earlier.

Dr. Bruenn told McIntire of FDR's heart failure and wished to proceed immediately to give digitalis to FDR. Both McIntire and a distinguished medical board that he appointed strongly objected to this course of therapy. This was another example of failure of the group to provide best medical care. But Bruenn persevered and became the advocate for his very famous patient. He had no other issues, political or otherwise, to consider.

He finally prevailed, was able to prescribe *digitalis*, and within a week FDR was greatly improved. Dr. Bruenn then became FDR's primary doctor and full-time cardiologist, and he would be by his side constantly from then on. Bruenn's appointment was McIntire's decision, and it was a good one.

Bruenn paid a price for his position, as he was sworn to absolute secrecy. As his commanding officer, McIntire ordered Bruenn to tell no one else of his findings, although it appears that Bruenn told Anna Roosevelt about her father. The cover up had begun and continued for the rest of FDR's life. Did anyone else know? No one knows for certain. Three people knew of FDR's diagnosis—Bruenn, McIntire and probably Anna Roosevelt. The members of the Navy medical board Drs.

James Paullin, and Dr. Frank Leahy also knew the diagnosis but kept their silence.[12]

It was well known that FDR was examined by other physicians at the Bethesda Naval Hospital and the Mayo Clinic. Their silence was maintained as a direct result of threats from the FBI not to reveal anything about FDR's medical condition.[13]

Since FDR's medical records are missing, one could speculate forever. The cover-up was somewhat effective. For reasons that remain unknown, Bruenn and McIntire never told FDR of Bruenn's findings and diagnosis, and FDR never asked. One could speculate that these events occurred in the era of keeping bad news quiet, starting with the patient. Only the doctor need be well informed.

FDR's marked hypertension would continue with blood pressure as high as 240/130. There was no specific drug treatment available in the Western world. Hypertension and stroke were the major sequelae. This was a silent killer. Rest, sedation, and salt restriction were the only available therapies in the West in 1944.[13]

The shrub *rauwolfia serpentina* had been used as therapy in India for over a thousand years, and a report published in English in the Journal of Indian Medical in 1942 showed that rauwolfia lowered blood pressure.[14]

This article about rauwolfia was cited in Index Medicus, an English-language medical reference that was available worldwide from 1879 until it ended publication in 2004. The index was first published by Dr. John Shaw Billings of Johns Hopkins, and was one of the major vehicles for the global transmission of medical information.

Maybe India could have sent some rauwolfia to FDR. In 1952, rauwolfia finally became available as the drug reserpine. It was the first drug in the West to successfully treat hypertension, but it arrived too late for FDR.

Was FDR really indifferent to his medical condition? About

thirty-four letters from FDR to his distant cousin, neighbor, and intimate friend Daisy Suckley, were found in a trunk in her home following her death in 1991. They are mainly filled with family gossip. But the following note did appear. FDR told Daisy that he knew he was sicker than the doctors were letting on. He wanted to retire but he could not do that during wartime. The soldiers and sailors were in for the duration of the war and so was he.[15]

In 1944, the public knew nothing of FDR's health. FDR was now disabled, not from polio, but from congestive heart failure. FDR had been dying under the care provided by Ross McIntire, who failed to note his florid congestive heart failure. If FDR appeared cyanotic (blue skin) when Bruenn saw him in March 1944, it is likely that the Democratic political bosses also saw this. The prospect of a dying president must have been terrifying for them. The Democratic convention would meet in June 1944, and the dying president would certainly be renominated.

The bosses feared that FDR would not survive a fourth term and that the next vice president would become president, sooner rather than later. They were never told the diagnosis, but acted upon what they saw, a very gaunt FDR.

The Democratic bosses detested Vice President Henry Wallace, so they dumped him from the ticket. They replaced him with Harry Truman, a Democratic senator from Missouri. The bosses were comfortable with him as VP, knowing he would soon become president. The choice of Truman was done in the "back rooms, shrouded by cigar smoke," with almost no public input. So much for democracy in 1944.[16]

The secrecy that Dr. McIntire orchestrated about FDR's health also concealed his own mistaken initial diagnosis, and his months-long failure to detect FDR's heart disease. When asked about FDR's health, he would say "it was OK." McIntire's denial cover-up would also serve multiple clients and purposes

1. It covered up his own failure to make a critical diagnosis of FDR's heart failure.
2. It provided cover for FDR's political fortunes vis-a-vis everyone else.
3. It provided cover for the Democratic party bigwigs who needed to keep FDR's health a secret from the American public in order to re-elect FDR and keep themselves in power.
4. Most important, FDR was the wartime leader of the Allies and McIntire's cover-up kept this information from the Axis powers. Such knowledge would have boosted German and Japanese morale and damaged Allied morale. With FDR at the helm, the alliance stayed intact long enough to defeat Germany and Japan, and to form the United Nations.

No mean feat. The Democratic Convention was in July 1944, and the Democrats had to make a decision soon.

IN FAVOR of FDR's nomination in 1944

FDR couldn't resign and retire from the war. His retirement would be a morale booster for the Axis. Keeping the Allied coalition intact became presidential job number one, and no other American politician enjoyed the international stature required to do that. The unconditional surrender of Germany and Japan and the formation of the United Nations were the goals of the Allies, and FDR was needed as the chief strategist for military victory and the architect of peace. On a more mundane level, another Democrat nominee was likely to lose a close 1944 election.

IN FAVOR of nominating someone else for president

The nomination of another candidate was based upon the

fear that FDR would die before victory and peace were won. FDR was not likely to survive a fourth term, and was so ill, he could die between the nomination and the election, thereby handing the election to the Republicans. He was physically unable to continue as commander in chief, and was not likely to be up to the job and could make critical errors.

How did the Democratic leaders respond to these hypothetical questions? They might have made a sports analogy. *Our best player cannot be kept on the bench when victory is so near. We can't worry about two or three years from now. The crucial time is now. Only FDR gets us victory and peace. He looks better since Dr Bruenn arrived on the scene. He may be badly wounded, but he has the guts and the charisma and the heart to get us over the goal line.*

And so, the 1944 Democrats rolled the dice and nominated FDR on the first ballot with ninety-two percent of the vote. He survived beyond election day and inauguration day, and somehow got the job done. Victory and Peace in Europe lasted for seventy-seven years. This was a great accomplishment for a dying man.

Senator Harry Truman won the VP nomination on the second ballot, after all sorts of voting shifts and shenanigans. The final selection of Truman remains a very convoluted and secret process that is still very difficult to process.

American voters were unaware of the seriousness of FDR's medical condition when he ran for a fourth term. Did the public have a need or a right to know? To dispel rumors concerning the president's health, FDR's advisors sent him out on the campaign trail in the fall of 1944.[17]

But the long campaign trail placed his life in danger. On July 29, 1944, after his re-nomination and before the election, FDR had a well-documented episode of prolonged angina while making a speech in Bremerton, Washington. Nevertheless, the campaign turned out be a political tour de force that show-cased FDR's charisma and oratorical skills.

FDR's speech about his dog, Fala, on September 23, 1944,

was a masterpiece of timing and wit and satire that skewered the Republicans. On October 21, 1944, FDR went on an eight-hour motorcade through all five boroughs of New York City in the rain in an open car. That was despite the heart failure and the recent episode of angina. FDR was putting on a full court press to win reelection.

But a very high price was paid...a Faustian bargain for the US. [18]

1. A very sick man was elected who would serve only three months of his fourth term.
2. Democracy was compromised by having FDRs illness kept from the public.
3. The next president of the US was not chosen by the people, but by a small group of Democratic political bosses who selected the next VP, knowing that he would soon be president. This would be the smallest presidential electorate in history.
4. FDRs trip to Yalta was an ordeal of 14,000 miles of travel in a wheelchair while in severe heart failure, a trip that probably hastened his death.
5. A very weakened FDR took on a healthy, vigorous Stalin at Yalta.
6. Vice President Truman was kept out of the loop and knew nothing about the A-bomb or any of the post war plans. Upon assuming the presidency, he was forced to play catch-up.

Truman and FDR had not met prior to the convention and would meet only once, for a photo op during the campaign. Since FDR knew he was very sick, his choice of Truman and his failure to keep him in the loop about the atomic bomb or war plans is inexcusable. Critics say that FDR's failure to include Truman is an example of FDR's diminished mental function. Dr. Bruenn said that was not so. He found FDR to be mentally sound. After FDR's death, the US wound up with an uninformed Truman trying to deal with Stalin and the Soviets.

Happily for the US and the world, Truman surprised everyone. He was a quick learner and did a great job as president, especially his first term. Note that Truman had no VP for all his first term, almost forty-five months. This may have been another impetus for the 25th Amendment.

In November 1944, FDR won his closest election, and in January he began his trip to Yalta in the Crimea. *"If we had spent 10 years on research, we could not have found a worse place in the world than Yalta,"* said Winston Churchill. How did the Allies allow this to happen? How could they subject FDR to such an ordeal? How did his doctors and friends and daughter allow him to go on this deadly mission?

Why didn't Dr. Bruenn veto FDR's overseas trips to Hawaii, Alaska, and Yalta? That was not in his job description and as a doctor in the military, he followed the chain of command, one way that Dr. McIntire kept control. Dr. Bruenn was too far down the political totem pole, he stayed in his assigned lane, limited to providing cardiac care. Approval of overseas trips for FDR should have been the domain of Dr. McIntire. But he did not have the wherewithal to prevent these overseas trips. McIntire's failure to stop the trip to Yalta was a dereliction of his duty as a physician. Bruenn could not bypass Dr. McIntire. He was under military orders, and McIntire was his commanding officer.

The conference could have been held in Cairo, or Rome or Malta or Stockholm or Istanbul, but apparently Stalin was afraid to fly or didn't want to leave the Soviet Union. Net result: a very sick FDR went to Yalta to arrange the post-war world. The Western Allies failed to obtain any significant concessions from Stalin before agreeing to go to Yalta in the USSR. This is very disturbing, now and then.

It's only 430 air miles from Leningrad to Stockholm, or 860 miles round trip. Compare that with FDR's 14,000 miles round trip to Yalta in the Crimea, which included traveling by ship to Malta in the Mediterranean, then by plane to Saki in Crimea, then a five-hour car ride for eighty miles over lousy roads to Yalta. How did Stalin get away with that? The war was still going on. The USSR was still dependent upon the US for military aid. We had some leverage with the Soviets; the failure to use it is suspicious and concerning.

Did FDR's ill health lead to a Soviet triumph at Yalta? FDR may have been too sick to resist the Soviets. He has been criticized for a poor performance at Yalta, and his opponents have said that this was due to senility or a stroke. Dr. Bruenn said that was not so, and he saw FDR every day at Yalta. He specifically stated that he saw no evidence that FDR ever had a stroke nor had any lapses of memory. But he described FDR as being greatly fatigued at Yalta. His color was very poor (gray), and for the first time Dr. Bruenn noted *pulsus alternans*, a sign of severe heart failure.

A very sick FDR was no match for a vigorous Joseph Stalin. The location of the conference in Crimea had been a big home field advantage for Stalin, who had a relatively easy train trip from Moscow to Yalta. The Soviets had a triumph at Yalta. The West got no guarantees for Polish independence and eventually abandoned its fighting ally, which was disgraceful.

Contrary to the Atlantic Charter, the USSR kept their territorial wartime gains in Finland, the Baltics, Poland, East Prussia, and parts of central Europe. The Soviets maintained their political power in all of Eastern Europe except for Greece.

At Yalta, the Soviets agreed to join the United Nations, and why not? They were to receive three votes (Russia, Ukraine, and Byelorussia) in the General Assembly, and a veto on the Security Council. They did agree to declare war on Japan within ninety days of VE-day, and they carried out this part of the agreement, but only after the US dropped an atomic bomb on Hiroshima.

FDR did all this travel in a wheelchair while in severe heart failure. The campaign of 1944 and the trip to Yalta are the stuff of heroes. The trip home from Yalta was even longer, as it featured a side trip to the Suez Canal to meet King Ibn Saud of Saudi Arabia. No president before or since has put it all on the line as FDR did in 1944-1945 when he gave up his life for his country.

March 1, 1945, FDR reported to Congress about his trip to Yalta. He looked like a sick old man and would be dead within six weeks. This was the first and only public sighting of FDR in his wheelchair. He also publicly revealed his need for wearing his metal braces.

On March 29, 1945, FDR went to Warm Springs for some rest.

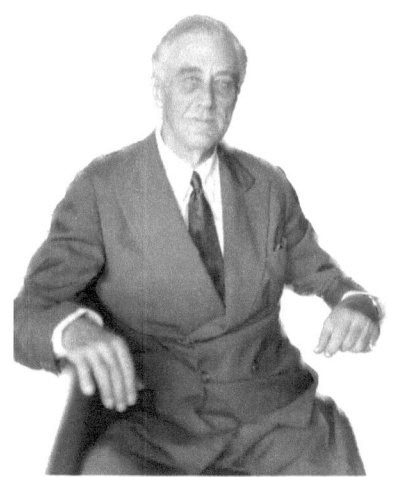

Image 15: April 11, 1945, the last photo of FDR, taken at Warm Springs, Georgia.

APRIL 12, 1945, while sitting for a portrait at Warm Springs, FDR complained of an intense headache, lost consciousness, and died. His blood pressure had been recorded at 300/190. A cerebral hemorrhage was the likely cause of his death. FDR was 63 years old when he passed. Dr. Bruenn was in attendance.

April 13, 1945, the cover-up continued postmortem. Dr. McIntire told the press that FDR had been in decent health and that his death was like "a bolt from out of the blue." All FDR's medical records are missing, presumably removed from the safe at Bethesda Naval Hospital; only Dr. Ross McIntire and the chief of staff of the hospital had the keys. No autopsy was done on FDR per the expressed wishes of Mrs. Eleanor Roosevelt, who was devastated to learn that Lucy Mercer had been with FDR at Warm Springs when he died.

If Anna Roosevelt had not insisted upon a second opinion, FDR might have died in early 1944 under the tender care of Dr. McIntire. That would have left us with President Henry Wallace followed by President Dewey or another Democrat, for better or for worse.

When he died in April 12, 1945, military victory in Europe was only a few days away. His military plans were in place and being carried out. On April 25, fifty nations met in San Francisco to write the UN Charter. This was FDR's creation and his legacy.

Apparently, at the behest of Anna Roosevelt, Dr. Bruenn wrote his first-hand account of FDR's illness in the Annals of Internal Medicine in March 1970. This article has been undisputed, authoritative, and accurate, and remains the classic account of FDR's cardiac disease and death. Bruenn referred to FDR's very large medical file which has since disappeared.

He admits there was medical information to which he had no access. But no one has seriously disputed his account of FDR's severe hypertension, heart failure, and death.

Bruenn's notes clearly state there was no evidence of senility or previous stroke. That has to be taken as the best medical evidence. But he describes FDR at Yalta as being greatly fatigued, with a poor gray color to his skin. There are still several questions about FDR's health that may never get answered (i.e., anemia, weight loss, tremor).

The McIntire and Bruenn duo had pitted the man with the superior title or rank (admiral and surgeon general) against his more medically skilled junior. Remember this, FDR was kept alive for the last year of his life, by Dr. Bruenn, only a lieutenant commander. Thank you, Dr. Bruenn.

The Presidential Succession Act of 1947 and the death of Eleanor Roosevelt are topics that can be found in the end notes [18, 19, 20, 21]. *They are of great interest but they are a digression from our tapestry. ELG*

16
"HOW IKE BEAT HEART DISEASE AND HELD ONTO THE PRESIDENCY"

On September 24, 1955, President Eisenhower, aged 64, had a heart attack at the home of his mother-in-law in Denver. This episode became a landmark on the path leading to the modern care of coronary disease. There was no cover-up surrounding Eisenhower's heart attack. There was actually a public display of Eisenhower's cardiac care. The purpose was to showcase the revolution in cardiac care taking place at Eisenhower's bedside. Eisenhower became the ideal patient and returned to an active life. Millions of Americans followed him returning to work, the marital bedroom, and the golf links.

Dwight David Eisenhower had a complex and interesting medical history. All of the six living Eisenhower boys were called Ike by their classmates, and they grew up in Abilene, Kansas, a bucolic small town where Eisenhower had an idyllic childhood. However, at age 16, he had a very dramatic and unusual illness, developing a severe infection of his right leg that had turned black.[1] Before he lapsed into a coma, he pleaded with his older brother not to let them amputate his leg.

He survived without amputation or antibiotics. This is well documented and almost impossible to explain.

Gangrene and sepsis with a spontaneous cure is very unusual. Ike's leg infection was one of those events that seem so extraordinary as to defy logic and reason. We just don't know what happened. Nevertheless, Ike recovered from this leg infection and went on to West Point and destiny. During World War II, he always remembered other farm boys from Kansas were going overseas into combat. This was his first concern.

Ike graduated from West Point in the class of 1915, a class that produced many future generals. Shortly thereafter, he began to smoke cigarettes. By the time he was appointed commander of US forces Europe in 1942, he was a chain smoker, consuming four packs per day.

From the 1920s to the 1950s, Eisenhower had multiple episodes of undiagnosed abdominal pain. In 1923 he underwent an appendectomy for one of these episodes. These episodes would later turn out to be *Crohn's* disease, a chronic inflammatory bowel disease that was first described in 1932 and not diagnosed in Eisenhower until 1956. This long delay in making a diagnosis was not unusual for Crohn's disease. [2]

How did Ike go from Abilene, Kansas to Supreme Allied Commander, defying death as a teenager with gangrene, having a moribund military career without any combat experience, and being stuck in the backwaters of Manila? For sixteen years he was bypassed for promotion and was ready to resign from the Army until World War II began in 1939.[3]

And yet, in 1943, this unknown officer became the Supreme Allied Commander in Europe. Ike's meteoric rise from obscurity to command bypassed many senior officers and was not unlike the legend of the unknown Arthur, removing Excalibur from the rock to become king. In four years, Eisenhower went from a desk job in Manila to become the most powerful military person in the Western world. However, Ike worked hard, was well like by fellow officers and had outstanding mentors like Generals Fox Connor and Douglas MacArthur

To paraphrase Tolstoy, Eisenhower did not appear to have been in the saddle of his destiny. Instead, destiny appears to have plucked him from obscurity amid the whirlwind of World War II to lead the Allied nations to victory in Europe.[4]

Eisenhower did in fact lead Allied armies to victory in Europe, managing an uneasy partnership with the Soviets, British, and French, and an almost impossible relationship with the British General Montgomery. Ike also managed the complicated battle lines at the end of combat in World War II in Europe, avoiding a military confrontation with the Soviets. Ike had the right stuff.

During WWII, penicillin became readily available for US troops. It helped prevent acute *rheumatic fever* which was epidemic during WWII. Penicillin was also used to treat *syphilis* and *bacterial endocarditis*. All three diseases may cause severe heart disease.

In another gift of military medicine, US military surgeons began to operate successfully upon soldier's hearts which represented a big breakthrough.[5] Until then, cardiac surgery was almost always fatal. Open heart surgery for the general population was coming soon.

After World War II was over, Ike resigned his Army commission in 1948 and became president of Columbia University. That same year the Framingham Heart Study demonstrated the association of diabetes, cigarette smoking, hypertension, high cholesterol individually and collectively as causes of cardiac death. And Ike quit smoking cold turkey because of one of his doctors advised that after reading some early reports.

Two new and very different medical therapies arrived on the scene in 1952 in the US. The ultra-modern high-tech heart-lung machines were first used for cardiac surgery. They would be joined by reserpine (rauwolfia), the first effective medicine to treat hypertension in the West. Recall that it had been in use in India for at least a thousand years.

In 1997, Clarence Lasby wrote a book titled *How Ike Beat Heart Disease and Held onto the Presidency*. Much of the following account is based on that book and the book review that appeared in the *New England Journal of Medicine*. Lasby described how this heart attack affected the president and affected the politics of his reelection campaign in 1956. Most significantly it changed forever the public perception of heart attacks. The lives of millions would change because of one man's heart attack. No other president's health had such an impact upon the lives of his fellow citizens. Furthermore, Ike became a model of personal involvement in one's cardiac care, which led to a great change in American behavior.

Eisenhower began his first term as president of the US in January 1953. His myocardial infarction began on Friday, September 23, 1955, while he was playing golf in Denver.[6] At first, he attributed his discomfort to the hamburger he had for lunch. He returned to the home of his mother-in-law, Mrs. Doud, in Denver, Colorado.

He continued to have what he thought was intermittent "indigestion" and went to sleep. He awoke around 2 a.m. with severe chest pain. His wife, Mamie, called Eisenhower's physician, Major General Howard Snyder. He arrived promptly and prescribed the following: morphine, papaverine, hot water bottles, milk of magnesia, and when all else failed, he instructed Mamie to sleep in bed with Ike.

Dr. Snyder had cared for Ike through many episodes of the undiagnosed inflammatory bowel disease and thought that this episode was more of the same. Snyder's therapy appeared to be working and Eisenhower soon fell asleep.

Several hours later, when he awoke a second time, Ike had another episode of chest pain, which was twelve hours after the first attack. Only then did Snyder call Fitzsimmons Army Hospital, and some army medics and a few colonels arrived with an EKG machine. It would show that the president was having an *acute anterolateral wall myocardial infarction*, a heart attack.

Lasby then described the comedy of errors of bringing the president of the US down the narrow steep stairs to the waiting ambulance below. Ike was then hospitalized in Denver at Fitzsimmons Army Hospital.

Dr. Snyder covered up his earlier failure to make the correct diagnosis by stating to the public that Ike had some type of gastroenteritis. There would be eleven different public statements to that effect during the first day.

To provide proper care for Ike, Snyder sent for Dr. Thomas Mattingly, an army colonel and chief of cardiology at Walter Reed, who would provide ongoing care for Ike, and would be in constant attendance.[7] General Snyder and Colonel Mattingly developed a similar relationship as had Admiral McIntire and Lieutenant Commander Bruenn. Dr. Mattingly was ordered to not criticize the care at Mrs. Doud's home, and to assume primary care for Ike's heart attack. So similar to Doctors McIntire and Bruenn.

Was it not reasonable for Dr. Snyder to assume that the episode at Mrs. Doud's is one more bout of the many episodes of indigestion that Ike had suffered for the previous 30 years? Before 1921, acute indigestion was listed as the number one cause of death in the US. Many cases had in fact been unrecognized myocardial infarctions. It all began to change in 1912. In a classic article in *JAMA*, Dr. James Herrick, a Chicago internist, stated the following: "Myocardial infarction (MI) was previously described as an autopsy finding that occurred only after death."[8]

Herrick declared that MI was not just a postmortem finding, but was very common during life as a distinct clinical event that was not always fatal. Many people survived their MI. *Coronary artery thrombosis,* seen at autopsy, was also present during life and was the cause of myocardial infarction, abbreviated as

MI and called a heart attack in common parlance, yet all three being the same.

Acute myocardial infarction began to appear as the cause of death on more death certificates and in 1921 took over first place, where it has remained for one hundred consecutive years.

The careful physician believes that one must always think of the most acutely severe illness that is likely to kill your patient. And since 1921, that diagnosis had usually been acute myocardial infarction, which is relatively easy to diagnose with an EKG. It is a very common disease, and so the utility of doing an EKG is very high. Dr. Snyder's failure to do an EKG for twelve hours was inexcusable.

He failed to consider the major threat to Eisenhower's life. Since 1921, severe anterior chest pain in a 64-year-old man is a myocardial infarction until proven otherwise. Doing an EKG is mandatory and needs to be done immediately. Dr. Snyder got caught in the trap of excessive familiarity with the patient. He was too close to the trees to see the forest. Again, so similar to McIntire.

Presidential Press Secretary Jim Hagerty arrived the next day, and Ike put him in charge of communication and told him to tell the truth, the whole truth and conceal nothing. People liked Ike for good reason!

Ike had insisted that the public be informed of his heart attack to avoid the deception of presidential health that had occurred with Cleveland, Wilson, and FDR. For the first time since Garfield's assassination, the public was informed of the condition of their sick president.[2] Unfortunately, that included the quality of his bowel movements. That information was quickly removed from future health bulletins. Upon receiving the news of Ike's heart attack, the New York Stock Exchange lost $14 billion on September 26, 1955. At the time, this was the biggest one-day loss, but the market quickly recovered.

Once again, a president suffered from a plethora of doctors;

at least five doctors were involved with Ike and each with a somewhat different agenda. There were three major players—Dr. Snyder, whom we have already discussed, Dr. Thomas Mattingly from Walter Reed Army Medical Center (formerly Walter Reed General Hospital), and Dr. Paul White from the Massachusetts General Hospital. Dr. Thomas Mattingly, a career army medical officer, became the man in the middle. Mattingly had some problems with his superior officers, who were not happy with a colonel in charge. But Ike felt Mattingly was the only one telling him the truth.

Ike's favoring of Mattingly made his superiors even less pleased.

A Dr. Leedham had told Dr. Mattingly that he had treated Ike for an MI at an army hospital in Augusta, Georgia in April 1949, an event that was not well documented. During that episode Ike collapsed and was transferred to Key West, Florida. There is no definitive record of this, which is curious, since, at the time, Ike was one of the most famous men in the world.

Dr. Mattingly spent a lot of time trying to figure out what happened during that 1949 illness. He thought it had been a heart attack. Dr. Mattingly found one of Eisenhower's EKGs from 1949. Initially read as abnormal, it may have shown *early repolarization,* a normal variant. These EKG changes may be difficult to interpret. In fact, all of Eisenhower's medical events from Augusta and Key West in 1949 are confusing. We don't know what to make of them.

Mattingly also thought that Ike had a *ventricular aneurysm,* the only doctor to think that. An aneurysm would significantly worsen Ike's prognosis. Mattingly thought the public would be best served by involving a civilian doctor. He asked for his mentor, Dr. Paul D. White of Massachusetts General Hospital, who agreed to go to Denver and consult on the case. Many felt that White was the ultimate expert.

In September 1955, the only effective treatments for an MI were morphine for pain relief, rest, and sedation for general comfort. Anticoagulants were of dubious value. There was nothing specific. There was no coronary bypass surgery, no angioplasty, no stents, no beta-blocker drugs, no defibrillators, no *thrombolytic* drugs, no coronary care units. Looking upon Snyder's performance from space, one might argue that his failure to do an EKG did not matter very much in 1955. There was hardly any useful therapy for acute myocardial infarction, so not much was lost.

Heart attack patients were treated in hospital with weeks of strict bed rest, resulting in a 65 percent survival for the first 30 days. Most surviving patients became invalids and never returned to work; their productive life was pretty much over.

On or about September 30 as Dr. White was arriving, Ike had a recurrence of his chest pains. There was no consensus among his doctors as to what was happening; pericarditis vs extension of the infarct, which may be a difficult diagnostic problem. This highlighted the lack of agreement on other issues. Ambulate or not? Chair rest vs bed rest? Anti-coagulation or not? How long to stay in hospital? Stay in Denver or go to Walter Reed?

Eisenhower and his team did not make public these differences of medical opinion. The public might only become confused by all these details, just as the doctors themselves appeared to be. In truth, many of the issues revolving around Eisenhower's care were the same that cardiologists were wrestling with every day worldwide.

How would the public interest be best served? Full disclosure or not? Many physicians believe that preliminary discussions should be private and privileged, especially when the diagnosis is uncertain. They reason that public disclosure might stifle a free exchange of ideas among the doctors who were searching for the truth.

But if Ike was running for a second term, should the public know all the facts?

In fact, who represented the public in these discussions?

Opinions are not necessarily facts. It is the public's knowledge of the doctors' consensus, and their conclusions that is critical, and not the rehashing of the differential diagnosis.

"Wasn't Ike entitled to *some* privacy?" However, Ike seemed ready to surrender much of his privacy in order to inform the public. Eisenhower had arrived at hospital at the tipping point of cardiology treatment, from a passive posture to an active one for patient and doctor. Dr. White was a leading advocate for this active plan.

Paul Dudley White was the ultimate expert. His presence was very reassuring for the public and gave enormous publicity to the significance of heart disease. He was a strong proponent for liberating the coronary patient from a life of invalidism. Advising the president to continue with his political career was in keeping with this philosophy. He was a proponent of early ambulation, benefits of exercise, and overall optimism. Contrary to his friend, Dr. Mattingly, Dr. White felt there was no aneurysm and there had been no previous infarct.

White was an outsider, the only non-military physician in the group, and he annoyed Eisenhower by going outside the military chain of command. He was too familiar; he even invited himself to lunch. Most significantly, he involved himself in politics and tried to get Eisenhower to resign and become an ambassador of world peace. This recommendation was not based upon Eisenhower's medical status.

Ike thought this proposal was way out of bounds, as do most historians. White brought no special diplomatic expertise to the table. His advice was uncalled for. White seemed to enjoy the limelight a bit too much, which may have been the real bone of contention between Eisenhower and White (i.e., who was top dog, the star?).

Many Americans have negative feelings about scientists and/or physicians who speak beyond their area of expertise, sometimes having an opinion on almost everything. How was Dr. White qualified to suggest that Eisenhower become a world ambassador for peace? Doesn't making that suggestion sully his overall reputation? Maybe Dr. Bruenn had his great success with FDR because he stayed in his lane and did not stray into politics.

Dr. Mattingly was the only physician who felt Ike should not run for a second term because of heart disease, but he never told this to Ike. He had spent his career in the army and respected the chain of command and went along with the decision to be announced later on by Dr. White. He would continue to go along with official recommendations and remain silent, except for the one time when he told Ike he had a 50 percent chance of surviving five years following a heart attack. Once again note the similarity between FDR and Eisenhower. Dr. Bruenn did not completely confide to FDR, nor did Dr. Mattingly reveal all to Eisenhower.

Meanwhile, Dr. Snyder had failed to keep adequate control of Ike's anti-coagulation therapy and Mattingly had to take over that task and correct it. After seven weeks in the hospital, Eisenhower left Denver on November 11 and returned to his farm at Gettysburg. He recuperated there before returning to work. He was a model patient, and by example became the role model for the active participation of patients in their recovery from heart attack.

Following Dr. White's plan, he took control of his own health by managing his diet to maintain healthy body weight and cholesterol levels. He took part in a regular exercise program, complemented with regular periods of rest. Control of stress and his explosive temper was a work in progress. This became the standard of care for treatment of patients with coronary artery disease and remains the core of therapy.

Ike's heart attack transformed forever the treatment of heart attack, and that changed the public's perception of heart attack. Life could continue, with some modifications. Dr. White's revolutionary care became the standard of care. This became a *permanent* benefit for the American people and the world. The remaining critical decision was whether or not to run for reelection in 1956.

Prior to Ike's heart attack, survival of an MI condemned the patient to a sedentary life, frequently isolated in a back room. Instead, Ike was returning to the very busy world of the presidency. The fortuitous junction of Eisenhower and Dr. White returned heart attack survivors from out of the back room into the marital bedroom, back to work, and onto the golf links. This was one of the greatest changes ever in American behavior.

Many of these survivors became activists and demanded more research, advanced care, and more available medications. The lives of millions changed because of one man's heart attack

THE FACT that Ike liked to play golf and to show off how well he was doing was the image that stuck with the public. The optics were powerful.

Could Ike survive another four years in the pressure cooker of the presidency? Ike and the GOP operatives felt that he was the only Republican who could be elected in 1956. This was reminiscent of 1944 Democrats nominating FDR for a fourth term. Furthermore, Ike felt that he *alone* could lead the free world during the height of the Cold War, similar to what Grover Cleveland believed during the Panic of 1893.

Two camps formed over this question, each of which had strong participation from physicians and family members. Those in favor of running for reelection were Ike's wife, Mamie, Dr. Snyder, and Republican operatives who did not want to give up their meal ticket.

Against running for reelection were Dr. Mattingly (though not very outspoken), brother Milton, and son John. A disquieting combination of doctors and family members became involved in the political process. Who represented the public?

But who was supposed to represent the public during these meetings?

Dr. White appeared in both camps. He was a strong proponent for liberating the coronary patient from a life of invalidism. Advising the president to continue with his political career would be in keeping with this philosophy. On the other hand, White was also concerned that this progressive recovery program would be jeopardized if his famous patient had another MI or died during his second term. White's reputation could also be jeopardized. White was ambivalent.

Ike weighed the pros and cons and decided *for himself* to run for reelection. Lasby's insight was that Ike's reelection represented his personal conquest of heart disease. This would serve as the hope and role model for all coronary patients. He stayed in control, a very active participant in the decision-making process.

A press conference was held on February 14, 1956, involving all the doctors, not a typical forum to make political announcements. Paul Dudley White finally made a decision. He essentially anointed Ike as the next president when he said that Ike should be able to lead a very active life for the next five to ten years. He had no evidence to support that optimistic statement. Even experts can overstep their boundaries. Should physicians have so much political power? Back in 1956, Dr. Mattingly continued to remain publicly silent on this issue, reflecting his adherence to the power of the chain of command.

Consider the 1956 pair of presidential candidates, Eisenhower vs. Stevenson. Ike was older and just had a heart attack. Stevenson was younger and apparently healthy. The public knew that Ike had heart disease, but Adlai Stevenson's heart disease was a well-kept secret. He died of a heart attack in 1965, four years before Ike. Because of Stevenson's secrecy, the public was not able to make a fully informed decision in voting for president in 1956.

There was one more medical hurdle for Eisenhower before

the November 1956 election. During the spring of 1956, Eisenhower had recurrence of his chronic abdominal pains. This time X-rays were taken of the small intestine, and they showed that Eisenhower had *Crohn's disease* by revealing the classic *string sign,* an indication of bowel narrowing.

Snyder did not act in a timely way upon receiving this information. Eisenhower then had a bowel obstruction requiring surgery, and the diagnosis of Crohn's disease was confirmed. Snyder's failure to act promptly was unacceptable, and once again a president had less than best care.

Ike was elected to his second term in November 1956 and had no further episodes of heart disease while in office. But one year later, on Nov 27 1957, Ike had a very small stroke, with weakness of his right arm, lightheadedness, and some mild speech impairment. He had no therapy, and did not go to hospital, although he was examined by doctors. Most of his symptoms quickly resolved after a few hours and never recurred. However, Ike was left with a slight speech impediment that persisted.

This event was somewhere along the spectrum of transient cerebral ischemia where brain cells are only injured, to that of a small permanent stroke in which brain cells die. The slight speech defect persisted and became permanent. Eisenhower was concerned about the three major illnesses that he had experienced in a two-year period (1955 to 1957) and how they may have affected his performance as president.

Accordingly on February 5, 1958, he wrote a letter to his Vice President Richard Nixon.[9] Eisenhower stated that in each of his recent illnesses "*there was some gap* (of time) *that could have been significant in which I was a disabled individual, from the standpoint of carrying out the duties pertaining to the office.*"

Referring to his stroke, he was afraid about something "*that might incapacitate you (Ike) mentally, and you would not know it, and the people around you, wanting to protect you, would probably keep this away from the public.*"

Ike named Nixon "*the individual explicitly and exclusively responsible to make the decision to take over in the event that he (Eisenhower) ever became so disabled as to be unable to recognize his disability.*"

Compare this with the episodes involving the severe illness of Woodrow Wilson and FDR, and their failure to communicate with their vice presidents, Thomas Marshall and Harry Truman. Ike's letter to Nixon was repeated by Kennedy and Lyndon Johnson, who made similar arrangements with their VPs. This began the political process that led to the 25th Amendment in 1967. Eisenhower had made another great gift to the nation.

At the end of his presidency Eisenhower addressed the nation and warned of the dangers of the military-industrial complex. During his eight years as president, no American soldier died in combat. His mother, Ida, a life-long pacifist would be pleased.

In 1960, John Kennedy defeated Richard Nixon in a very close election. Eisenhower handed off the baton to Kennedy and went into retirement. Nevertheless, Eisenhower became very ill after leaving the presidency. He had another episode of bowel obstruction that required surgery. He had several more heart attacks. He spent the last eleven months of his life at Walter Reed suffering several episodes of ventricular fibrillation that required defibrillation.

Eisenhower rode along with the incoming tide of the great wave of progress in cardiology. He was a disciplined man who took full advantage of modern cardiology and was a good patient. Coronary care units were first built in 1961 and the enhanced role of nurses was recognized. They were authorized to defibrillate patients on their own initiative. This was a revolutionary breakthrough.

The US surgeon general of 1964 reported on the adverse effects of smoking and millions of people stopped smoking, including tens of thousands of doctors. Another great advance of the 1960s was the advent of beta blocker drugs, shown to be cardio protective, lower blood pressure, and to treat and prevent angina pectoris. In 1967, coronary artery bypass graft (CABG) surgery began at Cleveland Clinic, where Dr. Rene Favaloro was the pioneer surgeon.

Eisenhower died on March 28, 1969. The family agreed to an autopsy, which revealed an old ventricular aneurysm that vindicated Dr. Mattingly's earlier diagnosis. Based upon the presence of the aneurysm, he should not have run for a second term.

Since Eisenhower's death, the cardiac armamentarium has dramatically increased with many new surgical and non-surgical interventions directed at the coronary arteries. One such therapy had its genesis in 1929 when Dr. Werner Forssman of Germany passed a urinary catheter through a forearm vein and threaded it forward until it reached his heart. He then took a chest X-ray to confirm its location. This was the first *cardiac catheterization*. Following that, Forssman labored in relative obscurity until he won the 1956 Nobel prize in medicine for his 1929 experiment.[10]

There are hundreds of statistics that I could show, but I will show only one. In 1956 the in-hospital survival for acute myocardial infarction had been around 60–65 percent. In 2018, the in-hospital survival for acute myocardial infarction was 96 percent.[11]

Ike became the first modern president to release his medical records, and the first president to reverse a cover-up and reveal that he was ill with a heart attack. Ike was the first president to address the issue of physical and mental disability that required the VP to take over the presidency. For all the above, Ike deserves to be in the top tier of presidents. Perhaps more important, Eisenhower's response to his heart attack was a liberating force for millions of patients. He took control of his care and resumed an active life. This was the teachable moment.

His new army this time was composed of cardiac patients, who followed him onto the golf course and resumed their lives. They promoted research for new and better care. Along with them came the medical profession, for their ways were now changed. As passive patients were replaced by active patients, doctors also became advocates for this new active care.

17

THE AGONY OF JACK KENNEDY, JFK (1917-1963)

The Jack Kennedy legend ranges from fact to fiction, like a potpourri of half-truths, bravery, political posturing, and obfuscation, and served with an occasional red herring

17A. The search for the truth about JFK's health remains elusive since the Kennedy family has prevented his full medical record from being revealed.[1] Some 59 years after JFK's death, there has been only a limited release of his medical records by his trustees. The medical history of John F. Kennedy constitutes one of the best-kept secrets of US history. The reasons for the cover-up are unknown. Perhaps it is only done to protect the Kennedy brand.

The cover-up appears to have served no useful purpose. JFK was an elected president, a combat veteran, an ex-US senator, a married man with a glamorous wife and two children. Daughter Caroline most recently was US ambassador to Japan and Australia. JFK had a distinguished political career despite having several medical diseases, none of which were disabling.

He bore his pain and tribulations with great courage, and successfully led the US and the western world through the

Cuban Missile Crisis. His leadership was the decisive factor that avoided nuclear war. He was a human being, but not a saint. That he had trouble with his medicines is not surprising and was not a crime, and nothing for which he needed to feel shame. He stayed in the political arena to his great credit, despite having constant back pain.

Unfortunately, he strayed over the line when he started using un-monitored doses of amphetamines. The blame lies with Dr. Max Jacobsen, a licensed physician, and a public menace, and does not lie with Jack Kennedy who was his victim.

Many US veterans of WWII saw sexual enjoyment as their due payment for years of living away from home. Unfortunately for JFK, prostatitis and urethritis didn't care about his combat experience, as JFK seemed to have had frequent genitourinary tract infections.

His father, Joe, was not exactly the role model for chastity and fidelity. Joe was one of the richest men in America, a philanderer, and a Nazi admirer. To JFK's great credit, he did not grow up to be like his father. JFK cannot be blamed for the sins of his father. But yet, why does all the secrecy persist? It is the cover-up that is worrisome.

In 2002, the Kennedy trustees finally agreed to open the JFK medical records to Boston University historian Robert Dallek. The records were limited to the years 1955 to 1963, and only two days were allowed to examine the files. Dallek recorded his findings in "The Medical Ordeals of JFK," published in the December 2002 issue of *Atlantic Monthly*. The article is limited in scope, but assumed to be accurate.

This chapter attempts to use Dallek's article as a Rosetta Stone to unlock the mystery of a complicated series of events utilizing incomplete information, fragments, and third-party accounts. Dallek uncovered the following information about JFK's medical history:

- *Colitis:* Inflammation of the colon, since childhood.
- *Osteoporosis:* Since 1944, causing multiple spinal fractures and chronic back pain, leading to many unsuccessful back surgeries.
- *Polypharmacy:* Including amphetamines, testosterone, cortisol, and eleven others; ongoing
- *Adrenal insufficiency:* Since 1946, with several severe episodes, one which lead to coma.
- *Urethritis, prostatitis:* Recurrent episodes throughout adult life.

In April of 1931, at age 13, Jack collapsed with abdominal pains and had surgery for presumed appendicitis. It is not known if that was the correct diagnosis. In the pre-CAT scan era, many operations for presumed appendicitis turned out to be unnecessary. Since the 1970s, CAT scans have improved the diagnostic accuracy of most cases of abdominal pain, including appendicitis.

In June of 1934, Jack Kennedy complained of abdominal discomfort and his parents sent him to the Mayo Clinic in Rochester, Minnesota. The gastrointestinal and colon tests indicated that Jack had colitis, but it is not clear what exactly he had.

Colitis may have been used as a generic term for any type of gastro intestinal disease.

Was this *ulcerative colitis,* or colitis of *Crohn's disease,* or *celiac disease,*[2] or every day benign *irritable bowel syndrome*? No biopsy or X-ray reports are offered in Dallek's article.

Jack wrote letters to his friends complaining about rectal bleeding, weight loss, and abnormalities with his blood. He complained bitterly about having repeated exams with metal pipes. They were probably referring to a proctoscope or sigmoidoscope. There is enough information here to exclude benign disease. Jack almost certainly had inflammatory bowel disease with weight loss, an abnormal blood count, and rectal bleeding.

This colitis may have been the beginning of many of his later medical problems. Over the years we learn little else about Kennedy's colitis. Before the late 1930s, there was no specific therapy for colitis, of any type.

Every human has one pair of adrenal glands, virtually identical in all aspects. Each gland sits atop one of the kidneys (adrenal), and is divided into an outer shell or cortex, and an inner center or medulla. The adrenal cortex produces several types of *corticosteroid hormones* required to maintain life. They control the inflammatory process, sexual function, salt and water metabolism, energy production and conservation.

Scientists began to search for a medical therapy to treat inflammatory diseases, and in the 1930s they first tried a crude extract of the whole adrenal cortex. Later, extracts were more refined, and scientists were able to isolate and produce purified samples of adrenal cortex hormones, (corticosteroids) in order to treat inflammatory diseases.[3] The first one of these was *DOCA (deoxycorticosterone acetate)*. Therapy with DOCA became possible when doctors learned how to administer the drug in the form of pellets implanted under the skin.

DOCA was an experimental drug in short supply, but DOCA therapy for adrenal insufficiency was first reported in 1938 in *The Lancet*. DOCA was also used to reduce tissue inflammation and perhaps also to treat colitis. There is circumstantial evidence that JFK might have taken DOCA as early as 1937. Much of the experimental work with DOCA was being done at Mayo Clinic where JFK was a patient in the 1930s. JFK was in the right place and time in the late 1930s at Mayo to have received DOCA for presumptive diagnosis of colitis.

While he was a freshman at Harvard, 1936–37, he wrote to his father worrying about getting a prescription filled in Cambridge, Massachusetts. "Ordering stuff here very [illegible word]," he wrote. "I would be sure you get the prescription some of that stuff as it is very potent..." Given that corticosteroids had just become clinically available and were being touted as a therapeutic cure-all, it is reasonable to speculate that the prescription JFK asked for was DOCA.

In 1938, JFK began having pain in the right sacroiliac joint of his lower back. No further description was given by Dallek. The pain could be due to mechanical stress. Another cause could be unilateral inflammatory disease of the right sacroiliac joint. It occurs in association with other forms of chronic inflammatory arthritis, i.e. Crohn's disease, ankylosing spondylitis, infections and psoriatic arthritis.

In 1943, JFK served as a US naval officer commanding a torpedo boat, PT 109, in the Solomon Islands in the south Pacific. The men on PT 109 saw no evidence of health issues, except for his chronic back pain which he took care of by wearing a "corset" and sleeping with a plywood board under his mattress. This sounds ordinary and mundane.

On August 2, 1943, PT109 was rammed by a Japanese destroyer and two men died in the resulting explosion. JFK and eleven other survivors spent about 12 hours clinging to the slowly sinking boat. They then swam to a nearby island 3.5 miles away. JFK towed a wounded shipmate by holding the strap of the wounded man's life jacket between his teeth.

But that was only the beginning. JFK swam back and forth among the chain of islands looking for food, water, and a means of rescue. That he succeeded in all three was a mark of his great endurance, courage, intelligence, and skill as a swimmer. All the men who went into the water with JFK survived.

Reading the account of these exploits in *Prologue Magazine* of the National Archives is eye opening. It is truly the stuff of super heroes.[5] It is unlikely anyone with any degree of adrenal gland disease or dysfunction could accomplish what JFK did in August 1943. Being shipwrecked would have been an enormous stress to his adrenal glands. Was JFK taking steroids (DOCA) while in the South Pacific? If so, how did he get a supply of DOCA in a combat zone? We can only speculate.

In 1944, JFK was discharged from the navy with a diagnosis

of osteoporosis, unusual for a 27-year-old man. This piece of hard evidence needs to be explained. The DOCA treatments he may have received as a young man for his intestinal ailments could have worsened and perhaps even caused both the adrenal insufficiency and the spinal osteoporosis that plagued him later in life.

This is a good example of Occam's razor, which is widely used in medical decision making. Occam's razor advises to seek the most economical solution. In layman's terms, the simplest explanation is usually the best one. Occam's razor is often stated as an injunction not to make more assumptions than you absolutely need. The razor cuts off the un-necessary bits.

Circumstantial evidence placed JFK at the right time and place to have received DOCA as early as 1937. In 1946, one of his friends, Paul Fay, watched JFK implant a pellet in his leg, presumably DOCA. We don't know for certain when JFK's DOCA therapy began, except that he was probably taking it in 1946. Few, if any other medicines, were inserted as a pellet under the skin. There appears to be enough circumstantial evidence to infer that JFK was taking DOCA from 1937 through 1946. His adventures with PT 109 are beyond medical explanation.

Occam's razor postulates that taking DOCA therapy from 1937 through World War II for inflammatory bowel disease, explains most of Kennedy's subsequent ailments. He developed osteoporosis as a consequence of the toxic effect of DOCA on the bones that led to his many spinal fractures.

He developed adrenal insufficiency somewhere after the 1943 shipwreck and before 1947. According to Occam's razor, this was a result of nine years of DOCA therapy with its erratic absorption, that eventually turned down his pituitary adrenal axis. This led to three well-documented episodes of acute adrenal crisis that occurred between 1946 and 1951. JFK still had sufficient adrenal reserve in 1943 to survive the events of the shipwreck.

Let's examine how this could have happened.

To provide answers to this question requires a short course in adrenal gland physiology, which is complex and complicated. Let's use a metaphor that has been presented several times before by others. Here is one version.

The endocrine gland/hormone system is like a large symphony orchestra. Assume you are listening to Itzhak Perlman perform Tchaikovsky's *Violin Concerto*. When things go well and the patient is healthy and the music is beautiful, all the parts are in perfect harmony. All the systems and instruments are finely tuned, and hormones and members of the orchestra are responsive one to the other.

Almost 200 years ago, Claude Bernard described this process that is now known as homeostasis. To create good health, all the parts of the body are responsive and attuned to one another. Like a musical conductor, the hypothalamus of the human brain receives signals from the internal and external world analogous to the sounds of the music. Is that sound soothing or jarring, loving or harmful, dull or exciting, obnoxious or beautiful? The hypothalamus is continually analyzing and responding to these signals with instructions to the endocrine system.

For example: save water, save salt, store energy, prepare for procreation, prepare for breast feeding, fight this infection, etc. When things are perfectly balanced, a state of harmony and good health has been reached. For the orchestra, beautiful music is made.

The orchestra is directed by the conductor, who has command of the entire performance. All the instruments follow his direction, as he listens to the sounds that are being made by the orchestra and compares that with his knowledge of how the music is supposed to sound. He is continually receiving input and giving instructions. The hypothalamus is the conductor.

Information is sent by signals. The musical conductor uses

his baton to send information to orchestra members, while the hypothalamus sends out hormones which act as messengers to the cells. The conductor waves his baton faster, the musicians play faster, now he wants to slow them down and he slows down his baton. There are hundreds of musical combinations occurring, as the conductor balances all the sounds being produced to make beautiful music.

In the same way the hypothalamus provides signals for more hormones. When the response is achieved, the system slows itself down. The hormones and glands respond to thousands of possible combinations of signals, always fine tuning, always responsive. The radio is always on, as the hypothalamus never sleeps.

What happens when a substitute enters the system? The substitute is never as good as the original. It may not be in harmony with other members of the orchestra. Or they may not know all the music. Or their violin may have limited range.

Another side effect is that the natural occurring adrenal corticosteroid is no longer able to respond to the conductor. DOCA has knocked cortisol out of its chair and out of position and it cannot see the baton to follow the instructions. It's as though Itzhak Perlman (cortisol) has been replaced by Izzie Perlman (DOCA).

Taking therapeutic doses of a synthetic steroid medicine such as DOCA for more than a few weeks can interfere with the entire system. The conductor and the violinist stop communicating and or stop responding to one another. And likewise for the pituitary gland (the first violin) and the adrenal gland.

In these patients, acute adrenal insufficiency could occur two ways. A sudden withdrawal of DOCA when the patient suddenly stops taking their medicine. The adrenal gland is unable or unaware of the need to replace cortisol, it is asleep. When there is a sudden demand for new energy, the hormonal system cannot respond with enough cortisol, and severe acute adrenal insufficiency occurs.

Because it was placed in the skin, DOCA absorption was erratic, and so was its metabolic effect. There may have been another complication of DOCA therapy. The chronic erratic absorption may have led to an unpredictable side effect to downgrade and deregulate the central controls of hypothalamus and pituitary. The entire system becomes less responsive in general, especially for an emergency. When the alarm is sounded, the metabolic response may be too low and too slow in arriving, and may be misdirected.

Despite his medical difficulties, JFK ran for congress in 1946 and won. Although he was taking medications for colitis, he continued to have abdominal pain and problems gaining weight. Continuous fatigue, nausea, and vomiting may have been the early symptoms of the as yet undiagnosed Addison's disease. JFK collapsed in London in 1947, and in hospital, he was diagnosed for the first time with Addison's disease. Kennedy was prescribed DOCA after this episode because there wasn't anything better that was available at that time.

Acute Addisonian disease or Addisonian crisis is a disease of all ages, sexes, and races that may present suddenly with profound cardiovascular collapse. Patients have many of the following symptoms and lab tests: severe weakness; pain in lower back or legs; severe abdominal pain, with vomiting and diarrhea leading to dehydration; and confusion leading to reduced consciousness or delirium. They may also have low blood pressure, hyperpigmentation of the skin, low blood sugar, and low serum sodium. Conversely, serum potassium levels will be high.

In 1855, Thomas Addison described a series of patients with many of the above signs and symptoms. They were all seriously ill and would die in a few years. At autopsy, many had widespread tuberculosis with involvement of their adrenal glands. The cause of death was destruction of the adrenal cortex cells that were producing the corticosteroid hormones, especially cortisol. In the 19th century, 70 to 90 percent of the cases were caused by TB.

The disease was not called adrenal failure or given a similar descriptive phrase. Instead, it was given an eponym and named after a famous person associated with the disease. In this instance it was called Addison's disease. The eponym stuck and most forms of adrenal deficiency are still called Addison's disease. Addison's disease is not tuberculosis of the adrenal glands. It is the eponym for any type of adrenal insufficiency.

Very few cases are now due to TB, nor have they been since the beginning of the 20th century when the rates of TB began to drop precipitously. The reasons for the decline are threefold: the work of Robert Koch in identifying the TB bacillus; the discovery of chest X-rays in 1895; and the sanatorium movement that isolated patients with TB away from the healthy but vulnerable population.

Today the causes of Addison's disease are *autoimmune disease* (70–90 percent), metastatic cancer to the adrenal gland, generalized fungal infection (i.e. *histoplasmosis*).[5] In fourth place is TB (7–20 percent). Another cause is suppression of pituitary gland function by years of synthetic cortico-steroid therapy. That was probably the case with JFK.

JFK apparently neglected to take his steroid medications on a regular basis. Accordingly, he had recurrent episodes of adrenal insufficiency with recurrent fatigue, nausea, and vomiting, and his doctors feared for his life.

During a trip to Japan in 1951, he had his final crisis of acute adrenal insufficiency. After that he agreed to be more rigorous about taking his medicine. However, by then oral cortisone had been produced semi-synthetically and was available by prescription. Medical cortisol was called hydrocortisone.

Because it was taken orally and not percutaneously, it was much better absorbed, more reliable, more effective, and safer than DOCA. Although it was a fixed one-time dose, it was much easier to take an extra dose when needed (i.e., the flu, broken wrist, a trial, an exam, etc.). No more pellets under the skin.

A normal life was now possible for patients. Preparation for major surgery and major accidents remained as major problems for management. Nevertheless, by 1951 JFK had his Addison's under control. Or so they all thought.

There was no longer any need to hide this disease from the public. This was very similar to a diabetic patient requiring insulin. Neither disease should diminish a candidate's election chances, nor should they interfere with presidential performance.

For whatever reason, the Kennedys decided to hide this from the public. Did they think JFK had TB as the cause of his Addison's disease, and that TB was unclean, an infection, something shameful? You cannot overestimate the sense of shame of 19th-century immigrants who contracted TB.

Did the Kennedys think that Addison's disease would mar the image of vigor they had created for JFK? There was no reason Addison's disease should limit his performance as president, and that should have been the message.

JFK did not get out in front of the message, acting as a role model, to inform the public of this great breakthrough of oral cortisone allowing a return to a normal life. Instead, the Kennedys hid behind a smoke screen of lies and half lies and obfuscation. This cover-up was not to be included in JFK's book *Profiles in Courage*. He did not risk his political career to do the right thing.

Eisenhower took a different approach for his illness. In 1954, Eisenhower benefited from the revolution in coronary care that was occurring during the acute phase of his illness. Eisenhower embraced this knowledge and shared it with the public, who followed his example of good cardiac care. Millions of people were able to resume a normal life. A great gift from the president to the American people. What confidence, generosity, magnanimity to share that information with the public. Eisenhower was following the US Army core values, especially selfless service. JFK was following his assigned task to pick up the mantle of his fallen brother and follow in his assigned path to become president. This was the credo of his father Joseph Kennedy, Sr.

By 1950 Kennedy was suffering almost constant lower-back aches from spinal fractures due to osteoporosis. He needed crutches to get up a flight of stairs. To attempt to alleviate the pain, JFK underwent multiple operations and hospitalizations in an attempt to gain relief. Despite all his surgeries, Kennedy's back pain was almost unbearable. X-rays showed that the fifth lumbar vertebra had collapsed. He had to rely on crutches more than ever.[6]

In August 1954, physicians from the Lahey Clinic in Boston recommended a complicated surgical spinal and sacroiliac fusion. They explained that without the operation, Kennedy might lose his ability to walk. On the other hand, the surgery was difficult and posed risks of a fatal infection because the steroids were suppressing his immune system. Despite the risks, JFK was determined to have the operation.

On October 10, 1954, JFK entered the New York Hospital for Special Surgery, but the team of endocrinologists and surgeons postponed the operation three times to assure complete metabolic preparation prior to, during, and after surgery.

The operation finally took place on October 21, 1954. It lasted more than three hours, and had only limited success. A metal plate was inserted to stabilize Kennedy's lower spine. But JFK went into a post-operative coma. The probable cause was, that despite all the metabolic preparations, Kennedy was having an episode of acute adrenal insufficiency. This was precipitated by the stress of surgery. Despite the prolonged pre-op preparation, Kennedy apparently had not received adequate cortisol preparation for surgery. How can that possibly happen?

JFK had received less than best care. We can assume that his pre-operative cortisol preparation was inadequate. This was in the days before the pre-operative check-off lists mandating that all the necessary steps for surgery needed to be ticked off a written list. This simple exercise followed the example of the pre-flight check list of the airlines and has led to a dramatic decrease in death from anesthesia and surgery.

JFK was finally treated with very large doses of intravenous cortisol and woke up after many hours in coma. All of this was described in an article in the July 25, 1955, issue of *Archives of Surgery*. Although the patients were anonymous, the authors were Kennedy's surgeons, his age was published and there is little doubt that in this article JFK is case number three. It showed that he had adrenal insufficiency both by history and as the outcome of surgery.[7]

But the article said that the postoperative coma was caused by a urinary tract infection. However, urinary tract infections rarely cause coma. In this case, it is alleged to have been severe enough to have tipped him into severe adrenal insufficiency. The authors might have minimized the serious nature of JFK's postoperative adrenal crisis.

With all the 1960 campaign controversy over Addison's disease, none of JFK's opponents quoted this article. Despite the lies and fabrications and smokescreens, the truth was hidden right there in the open, publicly revealed, and available but not quoted. The original medical records from the operation were not found by the surgeons who reviewed the case in 2017. Once again incomplete information leads to speculation.

In February 1955, another operation was performed at New York Hospital to remove the spinal plate which had become infected. Kennedy "resented" the back surgeries, which had brought him no relief and "seemed only to make him worse."

Because his prolonged absence from Washington could not be hidden, the Kennedys had no choice but to acknowledge JFK's back pain. Kennedy came through this surgical ordeal looking courageous because the public was led to believe his back pain was due to war wounds suffered on PT 109. This was not the case. JFK was not wounded or injured during the collision. He had a five-year history of back pain that preceded his shipwreck. Why exaggerate an incredibly heroic and truthful story? Nevertheless, his alleged war wounds gave him a hero's pass for walking on crutches.

As followers of Occam, we believe the culprit was DOCA and not the destruction of PT 109 that worsened his preexisting back pain. Why not say so? His endurance of great pain in fulfilling his political career is also heroic. We can admire him for that. Maybe it was the fear that a man on crutches could not win the presidency, although FDR seemed to manage that.

The Kennedys did not believe that coming clean about his other health problems would generate a similar result. The secrecy continued in order to maintain an image of vigor. All his other ailments would have presented a negative image,

From May of 1955 until October of 1957, Kennedy was hospitalized nine times for a total of 45 days. Most of Kennedy's confinements at this time were at New York Hospital, as he was treated for continuing back pains; a chronic abscess at the site of his 1954–1955 surgeries; repeated bouts of colitis; prostatitis urinary tract infections, and probable adrenal insufficiency.

Would the public elect anyone for the presidency with Addison's disease? Why the secrecy? By the time JFK was running for president in 1960, Addison's disease was no longer fatal and was readily treated with available synthetic medicine. There was no need to hide it.

Because of the secrecy, JFK may have missed doses of corticosteroids during his life. In order to keep up his energy, he resorted to the use of dangerous combinations of amphetamines and testosterone and increasing doses of cortisol. That is what the Kennedys needed to hide, the dangerous polypharmacy that led to a risk of increased aggressive behavior. There was no public acknowledgment of any of this.

JFK refused to let health concerns stop him. He managed to

hide all this from everyone except his doctors and intimate friends. It became the pattern that allowed Kennedy to pursue a political career.

To control his back pain, Dr. Janet Travell began to treat JFK with local procaine injections for muscle spasms in his left lower back. This began in 1954 and continued into the 1960s.

During the campaign for the Democratic nomination in February of 1960, JFK returned to his hotel in agony from back pain after spending hours in the freezing cold. JFK aide Dave Powers whispered to Kenny O'Donnell, another aide, "God, if I had his money, I'd be down there on the patio at Palm Beach."

Why was Kennedy subjecting himself to such pain? There are two responses to this question. Kennedy accepted the surgeries and the pain in order to fulfill his assigned role as the heir to the presidential destiny of his dead older brother, Joe. Deception was maintained at the potential expense of the citizens he was elected to lead. Was this was the motivating force that drove him to cover-up his disabling diseases, promote the myth of his vigor, shield his privacy from political operatives, and cover up any alleged illicit activities?

The opposite point of view is the following: the silence regarding his health reflects the quiet stoicism and bravery of a man struggling to endure extraordinary pain in performing his presidential duties. In retrospect, both motives could be in play.

Having said that, recall the presidency is not a hereditary position. It is part of a representative democracy. The consent of the people is a critical part of that, and that requires information about the state of the president's health. It is unacceptable for the president, his brother, or his doctors to lie about his health or to engage in half-truths and obfuscation.

JFK and his family have gone to great lengths to conceal his medical history. Before, during, and since his presidency, the Kennedys have guarded JFK's medical records from public view, apparently worried that even posthumous revelations about his health would hurt his reputation.

In 1960, during the fight for the Democratic nomination, aides to Lyndon B. Johnson, told the press that Kennedy suffered from Addison's disease. In response, the JFK campaign flatly denied that. In responding to the allegations, the Kennedy campaign used a narrow definition of Addison's disease. JFK's brother, Robert, said: "John F. Kennedy has not, nor has he ever, had an ailment described classically as Addison's disease, which is tuberculous destruction of the adrenal gland. Any statement to the contrary is malicious and false. ... In the postwar period he had some mild adrenal insufficiency, and this is not in any way a dangerous condition. And it is possible that even this might be corrected over the years since ACTH stimulation tests for adrenal function was [sic] considered normal in 1958. Doctors have stated that this condition might have arisen out of his wartime experiences of shock and malaria."

Bumgarner calls it "undoubtedly one of the most cleverly laid smoke screens ever put down around a politician. Adrenal insufficiency, no matter how caused, is a serious matter. The problem was life-threatening and requiring regular doses of cortisone." The main problems with Robert Kennedy's statement are JFK's post-war adrenal insufficiency can hardly be called "mild" given that he received last rites of the Catholic Church for episodes of adrenal insufficiency. He was near death several times. This was obviously a very dangerous illness. Even disease under control can lead to disaster during surgery, as in JFK's postoperative coma in 1954. By 1960, most cases of Addison's disease were not due to TB, to define it as such is wrong, a half-truth, an obfuscation, an attempt to deceive.[8]

The Kennedy campaign released a letter from two of JFK's doctors describing his health as "excellent" and Kennedy as fully capable of serving as president. Once again, a half-truth is offered up. JFK's health could hardly be excellent, unless you choose to redefine the word.

In addition, you do not need excellent health to be fully

capable of serving as president. See Andrew Jackson, Abraham Lincoln, Chester Arthur, Franklin Roosevelt, and Dwight Eisenhower.

Do physicians have any obligation to lie for their patient? What is the doctor's duty to the country vs duty to their patient? Let's recount the several physicians who had difficulty telling the truth about their presidential patient: all of Cleveland's sailor physicians, Dr. Grayson, Warren Harding's hotel doctors, Dr. McIntire, Dr. Snider, and now JFK's doctors.

In 1955, Eisenhower set the standard for truth that would have been readily available for Kennedy to pick up and follow. But the Kennedys chose duplicity and half-truths in order to deceive the public. This becomes another low point in our journey.

In the fall of 1960, thieves ransacked the office of Eugene J. Cohen, a New York endocrinologist who had been treating Kennedy. The thieves remain unidentified, but had a similar modus operandi to Nixon's operatives, so said the Kennedy camp. This put Kennedy on edge about the potential political damage from opponents armed with information about his health problems.

JFK's viewpoint was his collective health problems did not deter him from running for president; though they were a considerable burden, none of them impressed him as life-threatening. Nor did he believe that the medications he took would reduce his ability to work effectively. On the contrary, he saw them as ensuring his competence to deal with the demands of the office. The very positive experience with hydrocortisone that saved his life in 1951 solidified his positive reaction to the fact that he was taking medications.

The presidential baton was passed from Eisenhower to John Kennedy in what was a shaky transfer—the hotly contested, close presidential election of 1960. The electoral vote was 303 to 219 in favor of Kennedy. Texas and Illinois have captured our attention, since both states had a long history of election fraud. A switch of both states would yield a total of 270, enough to give the election to Nixon.

Nationwide, the popular vote was even closer. There was less than a 2 percent Democratic margin of victory in Texas, with less than a 1 percent popular vote margin in Illinois, Missouri, New Jersey, New Mexico, and Hawaii, where Kennedy received only 115 votes more than Nixon. Out of 68 million votes cast, the Democratic margin was 112,827 votes or a 0.17 percent edge.

Surprisingly, Richard Nixon graciously accepted defeat and refused to contest the election, sparing the nation months of turmoil and strife. This is one of the unexpected events in the very complex history of Richard Nixon. It has to be counted as a great defense of the peaceful transfer of power. Watergate is trivial compared to that, but the story of the president's burglars sold more newspapers. For our presidential ranking, this episode places Nixon above Pierce, Buchanan, Wilson, Andrew Johnson, and Trump. Detente with the Soviets and the opening with China must also place Nixon near the top tier of presidential ranking.

The Honor Code of West Point is "A Cadet will not lie, cheat, steal, or tolerate those who do." The ethos of Dwight Eisenhower left the presidency along with its occupant, and was replaced by sixteen years of Kennedy, Johnson, and Nixon. That era gave us the Cuban Missile Crisis, Vietnam, Selma and Birmingham, Kent State, and Nixon's impeachment. Do the Medicare and Civil Rights acts balance the scales?

Responding to a reporter's question the day after his November 1960 election, JFK declared himself in "excellent" shape and dismissed the rumors of Addison's disease as false. An apparent lie. Why do that? He had won the election and he was not going to be impeached because he had Addison's disease. Why continue the cover-up, which seemed to take on a life of its own? It is the cover-ups that sullied his reputation, not his Addison's disease.

During his time in the White House, Kennedy enjoyed a public image of robust good health that belied the truth. He was forever seen playing touch football at his home on Cape Cod. The mantra was vigor, pronounced as VIGAH.

Yet, according to the records of Dr. Travell, who became White House physician, JFK was under the care of many physicians, including an allergist, endocrinologist, gastroenterologist, orthopedist, and a urologist. Dr. Travell continued her local injections and JFK also received care from Vice Admiral George Burkley, the assistant White House physician.

Dr. Max Jacobson was an immigrant doctor from Germany who lived in New York City. He had made a reputation by treating celebrities with "pep pills," or amphetamines, which helped combat depression and fatigue. Jacobson, whom patients called "Dr. Feelgood," administered amphetamines and injections of painkillers that JFK believed made him less dependent on crutches. For JFK that image was critical.

In the 1950s and 1960s people knew less about the addictive power of methamphetamine. It was the prescribed drug of choice for weight reduction and pain (JFK took it for his back). According to the singer Eddie Fisher, also a patient of Dr. Jacobson: "Max with dirty fingers, pulling pills from his pocket to give to his patients. Not the doctor you want for the man with his finger on the nuclear trigger."[9] The president took Dr. Jacobson with him when he went to Vienna for a summit meeting with Russian Premier Nikita Khrushchev. Kennedy went to France, in June of 1961, to meet Charles de Gaulle. Unknown to Drs. Travell and Burkley,

Jacobson flew a chartered jet to Paris, where he continued giving injections to the president.

When the FDA expressed concerns about some of the ingredients in Jacobson's injection, they were dismissed by JFK saying, "I don't care if it's horse piss. It works." Secret care had led JFK to the tender mercies of Dr. Feelgood and methamphetamine treatment. Jacobson visited the White House 34 times in 1961–62, and made other visits to the Kennedy homes in Florida and Cape Cod.[10]

Let's hear from Dr. Raymond Adams, of Harvard Medical School. "The chronic administration of large doses of amphetamines may give rise to hallucinations, delusions, and changes in the affect and thought process, a state that may be indistinguishable from paranoid schizophrenia."[11] In 1975, New York State revoked the medical license of Dr. Jacobson for endangering his patients' lives with amphetamine injections. The records show he purchased over 700,000 needles and syringes during the eight years of 1964 to 1972.

Dr. Travell kept a "Medicine Administration Record" cataloguing procaine shots and the following oral medication: Lomotil, Metamucil, paregoric, phenobarbital, testosterone, thyroid hormone replacement, trasentine, penicillin and other antibiotics, Tuinal, antihistamines, Stelazine (though only for two days), amphetamines, and corticosteroids for his adrenal insufficiency, the doses for which were increased during times of stress. JFK took fourteen different types of medicine. Dr. Travell was continuing to inject him with procaine two or three times a day to relieve his suffering, which in the spring and summer of 1961 had become unbearable. In 1961, Dr. George Burkley concluded that the procaine injections, along with back braces and positioning devices which immobilized Kennedy, were doing him more harm than good.

In the fall of 1961, Dr. Burkley insisted to Dr. Travell that Kennedy consult Dr. Hans Kraus, an orthopedic surgeon. Kraus told Kennedy that if he continued the injections and did not begin regular exercise therapy to strengthen his back and abdominal muscles, he would become a cripple.

Burkley and Kraus used exercises, massage, and heat therapy to ease Kennedy's back spasms and increase his mobility. By January of 1962, Burkley and Kraus saw JFK having a better month than at any time in the previous year. At the end of February 1962, they described the past four weeks "medically speaking" as the most uneventful month since the 1960 campaign, and in April they pronounced his general condition "excellent."

Nevertheless, Kennedy continued to need extensive medication.

And here is the basic medical metabolic problem. A fixed dose of hydrocortisone can only approximate the body's need. To continually maintain his energy and vigor at times of stress, JFK resorted to testosterone and amphetamines in addition to increasing his hydrocortisone. Did the increased doses of hydrocortisone and testosterone and amphetamines make him unusually aggressive and combative? I keep asking the same question, because Dr. Adam's statement about side effects is disturbing.

Dr. Travell's records show that during the Cuban Missile Crisis JFK, took his usual doses of anti-spasmodics to control his colitis, antibiotics for a flare-up of urinary-tract problem and bout of sinusitis, salt tablets to control his Addison's disease and to boost his energy. Most significantly he also took increased amounts of hydrocortisone and testosterone and possibly amphetamines. Most worrisome were the major mental health side effects of these drugs.

Testosterone has a 10 percent incidence of increased aggressiveness, worrisome during a nuclear showdown. *Corticosteroid* induced psychoses are not rare. The unsupervised episodic use of *amphetamines* with its disturbing side effects of delusions and hallucinations, made risky behavior seem appealing. These are reasons they should never be given to a nuclear commander.

The Cuban Missile Crisis of October 1962, is a critical moment in the post-World War II history of mankind. When Dallek listened to the tape-recorded conversations from the crisis, he felt the medications did not impede JFK's lucid thought. On the contrary, Kennedy would have been significantly less effective without them, and might have been unable to function. Dallek also wrote that these medications were only one element in helping Kennedy to focus on the crisis; his extraordinary strength of will cannot be underestimated. Aggressive behavior is appropriate for a PT commander about to attack a destroyer, but not for a nuclear commander.

The US has a five-tiered defense alert system called the defense readiness condition or DEFCON. DEFCON 5 is the safest level with normal military readiness. DEFCON 1 is preparing to go to war, including the launch of nuclear Missiles. During the Cuban Missile Crisis, the US went from DEFCON 5 to DEFCON 2, one step from war or nuclear launch. How can the nation and the world be protected from such escalations ? Did Kennedy's drugs drive him to activate DEFCON 2?

The Soviets had a very similar five-tiered system. The Soviets never activated their system and remained at level 5 the entire time. Thank you, Nikita K. The only sane response to the Cuban Missile Crisis is total nuclear disarmament.

Many questions remain. Would JFK have been impeached if this drug use information became known, or would he have been sent for drug-rehabilitation under 25th Amendment Section 3, and or 4? Was JFK healthy enough to be president?

When Kennedy ran for and won the presidency, he was gambling that his health problems would not prevent him from handling the job. By hiding the extent of his ailments, he denied voters the chance to decide whether they wanted to share this gamble. Kennedy's charismatic appeal rested heavily on the image of youthful energy and good health and vigor that he projected. This image was a myth.

Ominously, President Diem of South Vietnam was assassinated November 2, 1963, only twenty days before JFK was shot. This set the stage for the last event in the saga of JFK.

17B. Assassination of JFK[1]

On November 22, 1963, JFK was assassinated in Dallas,

Texas. He was riding in an open-top convertible, sitting in the back seat with his wife, Jacqueline. John Connally, the Governor of Texas sat directly in front of him, next to his wife Nellie. VP Lyndon Johnson was two cars behind, riding with various federal agents. Both Connally and Kennedy were hit by gunfire at about 12:25pm.

After the shooting, JFK's car sped to Parkland Memorial Hospital, only a few minutes away. Parkland was one of the premier hospitals in the nation, and a major teaching hospital for the University of Texas's Southwestern Medical Center.[2] JFK was treated in Trauma Room 1 by well-qualified physicians. There was to be no repeat of Dr. Bliss treating the president on the floor of the train station.

Twenty-nine years later, on May 27 1992, the *Journal of the American Medical Association (JAMA)* published two articles. The first was an interview with the attending physicians at Parkland's emergency room (ER). The second was an interview with the pathologists who performed the autopsy at the US Naval Hospital in Bethesda, Maryland. These two articles were complemented by an editorial from Dr. George Lundberg, the editor of *JAMA*, a major peer reviewed-journal with a well-earned reputation of integrity and for publishing the truth. Much of the following narrative can be found in these three articles.

The Parkland doctors recalled that JFK arrived at Trauma Room 1 at about 12:30 pm and within moments all the critical staff were on the scene and in place. Trauma Room 1 was very crowded that day in November 1963, with medical and nursing staff moving about.

Everyone in the room had a different view of what was transpiring. Some were bystanders, some were primary actors. Several of the people in the room have written of their account of the day. It's understandable why their recollections may differ.

It is only the Parkland doctors' first-hand accounts of the

medical proceedings on that day in Trauma Room 1 that are of interest.[3] They described the following: On arrival, Kennedy had dilated pupils, was unresponsive, and had agonal (the agony of death) respirations. The right side of his skull was gone, leaving exposed brain, much of which had been blown out of the skull. There was spontaneous bleeding from the brain, which increased with the resuscitative measure of the doctors. The gruesome scene was magnified by Mrs. Kennedy walking about Trauma Room 1, holding in her cupped hands a piece of her husband's brain.

There were wounds in the front and rear of Kennedy's neck. The doctors wanted better access to his trachea for insertion of an endotracheal tube, so they enlarged the small frontal wound, and placed the tube in the trachea. Knowledge of this procedure did not make its way to the autopsy room in Bethesda, Maryland. Something else that did not make its way to Bethesda was JFK's clothing.

The consensus is that the tracheotomy/ intubation done at Parkland obliterated the original bullet wound at the front of the neck. That made it impossible to say if that was an exit wound or an entrance wound. Usually, entrance wounds are smaller and exit wounds are larger. Whether the initial bullet hole at the front of the neck was an entrance or exit remains an unsettled issue, and is the basis of many JFK assassination theories.

JFK did not respond to resuscitative efforts and at 1:00 pm he was pronounced dead.

This was about 25 minutes of resuscitation effort. There was no mention of whether he did or did not receive intravenous corticosteroids. Therefore, it was possible JFK did not get corticosteroids at that time. Such a shooting puts a huge stress on the adrenal glands, and it was not uncommon practice to give a large dose of corticosteroids, following massive trauma like this. It probably did not matter. JFK appeared to have received a fatal head wound.[4]

To summarize so far: JFK was rapidly taken to an appropriate facility where he received state of the art care by excellent clinicians. Their enlargement of the wound at the front of the neck had two results. It facilitated placement of the endotracheal tube, and it began a controversy of entrance wounds vs exit wounds that continues to this day.[5]

Garfield, McKinley, Cleveland, and Harding all suffered from their doctors' failure to apply the usual standard of care. The standard of care was and is to have the autopsy performed at the hospital where the patient died. If not in the same hospital, then at least in the same city or county. The physicians' duty to the patient continues after death and includes high quality professional standards of care and procedure, and respect for the dignity of the person.

The president deserves the best of care even after death. Autopsy doctors and pathologists have the duty to review clinical notes, patient records, and any X-rays or EKGs taken at the treating hospital. There is also the duty to speak with hospital doctors who first attended to the patient.

Apparently, none of that was done before JFK's autopsy, since the emergency medical care took place in Dallas, Texas and the autopsy was done in Bethesda Maryland. The pathologists in Bethesda, Drs. Humes and Boswell did not have the benefit of any of that Dallas information. Less than best care. How could that possibly happen to the president of the United States? It happened because the pathologists were instructed if not, in fact, commanded to hurry.

In June 1963, Dr. Earl Rose became the medical examiner for the city and county of Dallas. According to *The New York Times*, he was "hired by the county to establish a scientifically valid medical examiner's system to replace its existing system of elected lay coroners."

On November 22, 1963, Dr. Rose was in his office at Parkland Memorial Hospital across the corridor from Trauma Room 1, when he received word that Kennedy was pronounced dead.

He walked across the corridor to the Trauma Room1 to begin preparations for JFK's autopsy.

A strange moment in US history then took place. Dr. Rose was met by Secret Service Agent Roy Kellerman and Kennedy's assistant personal physician, Vice Admiral George Burkley, who told him there was no time for an autopsy because Mrs. Kennedy would not leave Dallas without her husband's body, and Lyndon Johnson would not leave Dallas without Mrs. Kennedy, and they were leaving immediately.[6] This was based on the questionable assessment of the Secret Service that the presidential entourage could not safely remain in Dallas, and had to leave in a hurry.

At the time of the assassination of Kennedy, the murder of a United States president was not under federal jurisdiction.[7] Dr. Rose objected, insisting that Texas law required him to perform a post-mortem examination prior to the removal of the body. A heated exchange ensued as he argued with Kennedy's aides. Kennedy's body was placed in a casket and then onto a gurney. Accompanied by Mrs. Kennedy and Vice Admiral Burkley, it was rolled down the corridor. Backed by a policeman, Dr. Rose stood in the hospital doorway in an attempt to prevent the removal of the coffin. The president's widow was forcefully removing her husband's body from the hospital and absconding with him to Washington, DC.

In an interview with the *Journal of the American Medical Association* in 1992, Dr. Rose stated that after the heated exchange with the Secret Service and Burkley, he stepped aside feeling that it was unwise to exacerbate the tension. There are multiple reports that Dr. Rose was held at gunpoint as the Kennedys left the hospital. When asked about the gunpoint incident in 1992, Dr. Rose replied, "that might have happened, I'm not sure."

Rose observed, "The law was broken" and that "[a] Texas autopsy would have assured a tight chain of custody on all the evidence." Dr. Rose believed he and his staff should have been allowed to perform the post-mortem examination of Kennedy;

if he had, the many conspiracy theories about the assassination would have been quelled.[8] Kudos to Dr. Rose, standing up for the right thing for the right reasons.

The Kennedys paid a high price for willfully breaking the laws of Texas. Instead of doing the autopsy right away and delaying the departure of the presidential party for a few hours, the Kennedys opened the door for many of the conspiracy theories that followed. Their high-handed behavior in breaking the laws of Texas and using force to accomplish that, set the stage for the belief that something was not quite right. It seemed unusual to fly from Dallas with the president's body. The entire assassination was now stained by a certain sense of irregularity. All of this began on day one.

After JFK was pronounced dead at 1 p.m., Vice Admiral George Burkley became a man in a hurry. He promoted political expediency, removing the body immediately from Parkland to do the autopsy at Bethesda Naval Hospital and not the world-famous Armed Forces Institute of Pathology (AFIP), Silver Springs, Maryland, and to perform the autopsy immediately upon arrival. The choice of Bethesda was Mrs. Kennedy's. Since Jack served in the navy during World War II, she wanted his autopsy to be done at a naval hospital. What is the reason for the rush? JFK was dead. This was the president; accuracy and thoroughness should be the main concern. The need for speed was not necessary.

JFK's body was placed in a heavy bronze casket and taken to Love Field in Dallas, and onto Air Force One with considerable difficulty, requiring the removal of partitions from the interior of the presidential plane.

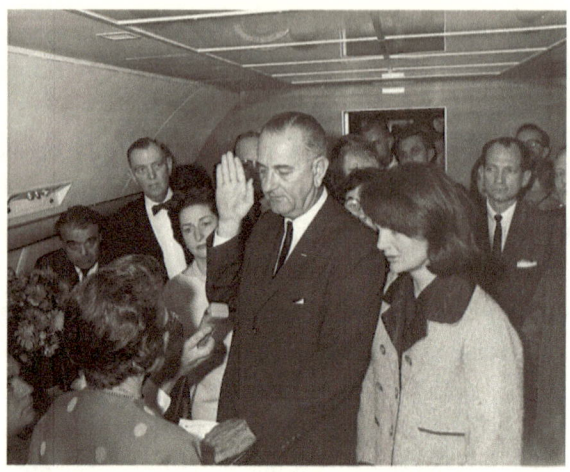

Image 16: LBJ sworn in as President Nov 22, 1963 onboard Air Force One, on the tarmac in Dallas. The grief-stricken Jackie Kennedy is by his side.

Lyndon Johnson and Mrs. Johnson, Mrs. Kennedy and other members of their entourage gathered inside the plane for the swearing in of LBJ as president of the US. The ceremony took place at 2:38 p.m. inside Air Force One, while still on the tarmac in Dallas. The whole process lacked a sense of grace and dignity. Why drag Mrs. Kennedy into the photo op?[10]

Why can't she be allowed to grieve in private? After the ceremony, Air Force One took off for Maryland.

Air Force One landed at Andrews Air Force Base, Maryland around 6 p.m. The rest of the itinerary included unloading the casket from Air Force One and transferring it onto a helicopter, flying to Bethesda, unloading the helicopter, and bringing the casket to the morgue via ambulance. That is one helicopter flight and four transfers of the heavy casket in about two hours Overall, there was not much time that the casket was left unattended; this was a tight time line. There had been little opportunity or time to interfere with the corpse. This is mentioned as we seek some explanation for the irregular, incomplete, faulty autopsy reports that will be issued. There is also a question about the accuracy of this timeline, since the casket arrived at

Bethesda about 20 minutes before Burkley and his staff.[9] The autopsy was to begin at 8 p.m.

Dr. James Humes was the chief pathologist at Bethesda with the rank of commander. He was instructed by the navy surgeon general, Rear Admiral Edward Kenney "to hurry over to the hospital." It was 5:15 p.m.

By the time he arrived at the hospital, he had heard the news from Dallas and was beginning to get the message that this was about the president's body. Once inside the hospital, Kenney told him "to be prepared to do an autopsy." Dr. Humes then contacted his associate, Dr. J. Thornton Boswell, also a navy commander, to begin the preparation. Both doctors were board certified pathologists.

Dr. Pierre Finck, an army lieutenant colonel, was a ballistic expert at the Armed Force Institute of Pathology, one of the world premier centers for pathological study. He was on-site to assist with the autopsy and to act as a consultant. Some of the criticism of the autopsy would have disappeared if the autopsy were performed at AFIP. But Dr. Burkley wanted to placate Mrs. Kennedy and acceded to her wish to have the autopsy done at Bethesda. Unfortunately, the bypass of AFIP raised more questions, and added more fuel for the growing number of conspiracy theories.

A large bronze casket arrived in the morgue, accompanied by Vice Admiral Burkley and a host of military officers in dress uniform. A naked body covered only by a sheet was removed from the casket, and placed upon the autopsy table. The pathologists noted all the clothing was missing. Gauze and bandages covered the head wound.

Was this the president of the United States? A body was delivered by military escort to Bethesda with no clothes and no identity (ID) toe tag. Neither one of JFK's brothers nor his wife came to the morgue to identify the body. Where were his clothes, his wallet, or his jewelry? Doesn't that strike you as unusual, especially since there are reports that Jackie placed her wedding ring on JFK's hand after he was pronounced dead at Parkland. How does a wedding ring disappear from a corpse?

The pathologists performed the traditional and unreliable "Looks like" test and stated they thought it was President Kennedy, even though half of his skull was missing. Do you think that one could make a positive ID on someone who was missing half their head, and had a very large hole in the front of their neck?

Nothing was mentioned about the surgical scars on his back. Nothing was said about the absence or presence of the usual ID toe tag. There was too much assumption and, perhaps, too much subconscious coercion by the military chain of command, who were present in the morgue in dress uniform.

In medical school we are taught repeatedly to "assume, nothing!" Assume is the ass that connects "u" and "me." Where was the independent questioning pathologist? Who speaks for the patient? Who speaks for the public? Who is this body? Where is the medical history? Who ordered the autopsy? Who will receive the autopsy report—the Dallas authorities or the Washington, DC police? The US Navy? Was there a coroner's inquest?

Where does that take place?

Recall that all the usual chain of possession of evidence was gone. It was only later on that forensic dentists were able to confirm JFK's identity by comparing his dental X-rays with those of the body in the morgue.

Vice Admiral Burkley continued his sense of urgency by asking the pathologists to hurry their exam as much as possible. After the autopsy was finished at midnight, he gave them less than 48 hours to finish their report. Remember they have not yet spoken with the Parkland doctors or reviewed the X-rays and photographs produced there. They did not have JFK's clothes, or his wallet, jewelry, etc. Speed prevailed for uncertain reasons. Why the rush? Fifty-nine years later, we are still waiting for an answer, why was JFK murdered?

Many deficiencies in the autopsy report have to do with the drive for speed, and the lack of information and communication with Parkland Hospital. But there were telephones available to speak with the Parkland staff, long distance phone calls having been in use since 1915.

As a young medical student, I helped perform autopsies at a city hospital in Queens, New York. It was drummed into me how critical it was to make the proper identification of the body and to follow that through to the final report. So many factors were impacted: the patient's religion, life insurance and workman's compensation, criminal investigation, discovery of hereditary disease, closure for family members, and follow-up information for the patient's treating physician. There was great interest in the postmortem exam of Kennedy's adrenal glands because Kennedy's apparent history (at that time) of adrenal insufficiency. There is no mention in the autopsy report of JFK's adrenal glands by gross or microscopic exam. They were just not mentioned. This is hard to imagine, because identifying both adrenal glands is a standard of autopsy reports. Sometimes it is difficult to find and identify the adrenal glands. My instructors always insisted upon a detailed description of the search for and the examination of the adrenals. This was at one step toward seeing that I had done a complete autopsy.

The medical student in me recoils from an incomplete autopsy performed upon the president. None of the surgical scars on his back were described. The skeleton and gastrointestinal tract were both described as normal by gross and microscopic exam. That was unlikely. JFK had inflammatory bowel disease since childhood and that would have been seen on the microscopic slides of the intestines and probably on gross inspection of the bowels.

He had osteoporosis of his spine since 1944 and had the external scars of multiple surgeries on his back and internal changes of his spine due to multiple surgeries. In addition, he had several vertebral fractures during his life. None of that was mentioned in the autopsy report. How was any of this missed?

Such an autopsy report raises several questions: Did they have the right body? The forensic dental exam said the answer was yes, the body was JFK.

In 1992, the pathologists at Bethesda responded to a long interview in *JAMA*. In retrospect this was a blockbuster.

- They did indeed examine both left and right adrenal areas in 1963 and only found tiny fragments of adrenal tissue. This was profound atrophy of the adrenal glands, but they failed to report that. *JFK had Addison's disease.* Why did the pathologists fail to mention that in the 1963 autopsy report?[12]
- A major piece of history had been hidden by the pathologists for 29 years.
- The pathologists were pressured unsuccessfully by the Kennedy family not to examine the abdomen, the location of the adrenal glands. The pressure of the cover-up had made its way into the morgue.[13]
- For whatever reason, the pathologists failed to mention the word adrenal gland in their initial report. That is inexcusable, much less than best care.
- Perhaps that happened because the pathologists were threatened with arrest and court martial if they made public any autopsy information. Another low point had arrived for American medicine.[14]
- The pathologists were instructed not to dissect the throat and neck wounds.[15] Why was that?
- The original autopsy notes were burned because there was some blood on them.
- No explanation was ever offered for the erroneous statements of normal intestines and bones.

This is the president of the United States. Does not he deserve the best of care? Does not history cry out for accuracy and thoroughness? How does this happen? Who can know?

All of these flaws may be due to doing things in a hurry, but the autopsy reports are so flawed that other concerns are possible.

Bypassing the AFIP located in Silver Springs, Maryland, only a few miles from Bethesda Naval Hospital, had opened up the issue of the credentials and expertise of the Bethesda pathologists. The doctors were initially criticized because they were not the pathologists at AFIP. However, the evidence shows that the Bethesda pathologists were well qualified and board certified.

But with so many flaws and irregularities in the autopsy report and process, it is the pathologists' credibility that became an issue. Were they coerced? We know they were threatened. Someone is playing hardball. But who was it?[16]

All of these questions and controversies came about because Mrs. Kennedy wanted the autopsy to be done at a naval hospital. She did not want to leave her husband and she had her way. And so critical information from Dallas, such as the tracheotomy, never made its way to Bethesda, or was forgotten and the entrance wound debate lives on in history.

When the Bethesda pathologists began their examination, they did not know that the Parkland doctors had enlarged the anterior throat wound to gain easy access to the trachea.

And thus began the 59-year-old controversy of exit wound vs entrance wounds, the larger wound is assumed to be the exit wound and vice versa.

ALL THE SYMPATHY goes to Jackie Kennedy, a brave and courageous lady. But please no more special rules for special people. Once again, special treatment for presidents does not guarantee the best outcome. Perhaps the Kennedys should have followed the example of Grover Cleveland and performed the autopsy on a boat cruising on the Potomac? That would have protected all their concerns for secrecy,

The story that the presidential entourage could not safely stay in Dallas for a few hours was unjustified. Who can tell where danger lies? On the return flight to Washington, DC, Air Force One had to fly at 50,000 feet to avoid a severe storm front, the first time the presidential jet ever flew at that altitude.[17]

Democracy abhors a medical coverup. Remember Woodrow and Edith Wilson. The incomplete, erroneous JFK autopsy was an attempt by someone to rewrite political and medical history to their advantage. The integrity of the autopsy system was threatened and that is relevant to medical history

The events of November 22, 1963, are etched in my memory forever. I was a 24-year-old medical student and was in the library, studying for exams in surgery. Peter S., another student, raced in and told us the president had been shot to death. I was devastated and in shock. There were six students on the surgery rotation, and we were summoned to the office of Dr. C. B. Mueller, the chief of surgery. He had been a stern, tough taskmaster so far.

To my amazement he softened and told us that he had been a poor country boy who had gone to school on scholarships. Becoming a physician was a privilege and an honor, and in return physicians were to do the best they could at all times, especially in terrible times like November 22, 1963. We were told to return to the surgical wards. Medical school continued. The following morning the six of us gathered to take written exams in surgery. None of us passed the exams. I guess, we were still in shock. We did come back later and pass the final exams.

The memory roll continues, the black-and-white TV pictures, all weekend, non-stop, Walter Cronkite's unsuccessful attempts to soothe us. There is no philosophy I know of that can respond to November 22, 1963. Writing about this episode is like a PTSD event, reliving the horror. I am left with a kaleidoscope of images flashing before me. Jackie on the trunk of the limo, Jackie at LBJ's swearing in, a smirking Oswald holding his rifle, Jack Ruby shooting Oswald on live TV, all the Dallas police with their 10-gallon hats, the funeral cortege in Washington, Dr. Mueller, and, of course, Jack Kennedy with the fatal gunshot wound to his head. The sense of horror and disbelief has not faded with time.

18

THE SHOOTING OF RONALD REAGAN, AND THE TRIUMPH OF US MEDICINE

His survival from a deadly gunshot wound represents the triumph of US medicine, especially the emergency response system. The fragile status of the process of transition of power was once again exposed.

Emergency services before 1980 were unorganized and chaotic; there were few, if any national standards of care. In the late 1970s, an organized system evolved with a comprehensive policy that included programs of public awareness, courses on Basic Life Support, training of first responders (i.e., police, fire, EMTs), and creation of a universal emergency phone system and network (911).

The policy stated that those first on the scene needed to call 911 and to immediately begin cardio pulmonary resuscitation (CPR). Emphasis was placed on the speed of delivery of care. In the case of a stroke, time saved was equated with the brain cells being saved. For a cardiac arrest, time saved meant saving heart muscle.

Ideal time limits were established, and faster response times were associated with better clinical outcomes. They were

60 minutes for trauma, 45 minutes for stroke, and five minutes for cardiac arrest. The time limits had some flexibility, and that meant that CPR did not have to stop at exactly five minutes. Longer times were allowed for younger children, drowning victims, patients with hypothermia, and drug overdoses.

Receiving hospitals were stratified according to their staffing and capability The criteria were strict. For example, to receive head trauma cases, the hospital needed to have continuous onsite presence of a neurosurgeon, a radiology team, a surgical ICU, plus necessary equipment and trained staff.

So, *triage* in the field to identify the most appropriate level of hospital care became the first critical decision. For example, head trauma cases should not be sent to an urgent care facility or to a small community hospital without neurosurgeons onsite.

The policy of rapid battlefield evacuation began in the Civil War at the Battle of Gettysburg and continues to the present day. That battle witnessed the beginning of a dedicated ambulance corps of men, wagons, and horses. During the past century, the speed of transport has increased from stretcher bearers, to horses and wagons, to motor cars, to jeeps, and to helicopters.

As the speed of evacuation from the battlefield increased, so did the survival rate. Because of the rapid evacuation of wounded soldiers from the front lines during WWII, over 98 percent of US soldiers who arrived alive at a medical aid station survived.

In addition, survival was also increased when medics began to treat wounded soldiers with rapid infusion of plasma right on the battlefield. This was due to the work of the Afro-American physician Dr. Charles Drew who created the blood banking system and promoted the use of plasma as emergency care in WWII. Sadly, he needed to resign to protest the racial segregation of the banked blood.[1]

During WWII, US Army surgeons routinely performed chest surgery, including successful operations performed on soldiers' hearts. Prior to World War II, there had been only a few isolated cases of successful cardiac surgery. However, during World War II, US Army surgeon Dwight Harkens removed bullets and shrapnel from over 140 beating hearts with zero fatalities. This was pretty amazing, since bullet wounds to the heart had previously almost always been fatal.[2]

Ronald Reagan was shot on March 30, 1981, only 70 days into his presidency, as he was leaving the Hilton Hotel, Washington, DC, by a side entrance and getting into his limousine. At age 70, he had suffered a very dangerous gunshot wound (GSW) to his chest. His survival had depended upon receiving superb medical and surgical care.

As Reagan was leaving the hotel, the shooter got off six shots before being subdued. Bullets struck Press Secretary James Brady, police officer Thomas Delahanty, Secret Service agent Tim McCarthy, and President Reagan.

1st bullet: Struck Jim Brady in the head.

2nd bullet: Struck police officer Delahanty in the neck.

3rd bullet: The shooter John Hinckley then had a clear shot at the president. Fortunately, Alfred Antenucci, a Cleveland labor official, was standing near Hinckley and saw him fire the first two shots. Antenucci then hit Hinckley in the head and pulled him down to the ground.[3]

Upon hearing the first two gunshots, Special Agent in Charge Jerry Parr pushed Reagan into the limousine. With Antenucci spoiling Hinckley's aim and Parr pushing Reagan into the limo, the third bullet overshot the president, narrowly missing his head. Hinckley got off three more shots as he was being taken down by Antenucci.

4th bullet: Hit agent McCarthy in the chest. Tim McCarthy had stepped in front of President Reagan, and took a bullet to the chest, but would go on to make a full recovery. While all Secret Service agents are trained to take a bullet for the president, McCarthy is the only one to have done so.

5th bullet: Missed and hit the limousine.

6th bullet: Also hit the limousine but ricocheted into Reagan's chest. It entered his left chest causing a collapse of the left lung and ended up 25mm (about one inch) from his heart, a life-threatening wound. All four gunshot victims survived, but Brady suffered brain damage and became permanently disabled. His death in 2014 was labeled a homicide because it was ultimately caused by this gunshot wound.

THE GOLDEN HOUR. If patients survive the initial trauma, medical personnel have an additional 60 minutes to resuscitate and save them. This was an extension of the battlefield experience of World War II. This concept was first described by Dr. R. Adams Cowley, MD at the University of Maryland Medical Center in Baltimore.[4]

From his personal experiences and observations in post-World War II Europe, and then in Baltimore in the 1960s, Dr. Cowley recognized that the sooner trauma patients reached definitive care, the better their chance of survival. Especially true, if they arrived within 60 minutes of being injured.

Just prior to Reagan's arrival at the GWH Emergency room, a surgical resident had inserted a chest tube in a patient and promised a medical student that he could insert the next one. (Remember. *"See one, do one, teach one"*)

T - ZERO. **START THE CLOCK.** Reagan is shot.

Everything happened very fast, but the Secret Service agents knew what to do. They sprang into action immediately. Secret Service agent Jerry Parr pushed Reagan into the limo and made the critical and correct decision to go directly to the George Washington Hospital (GWH). With the wounded Regan aboard, the presidential limousine sped off to GWH. The consensus is that Parr's actions saved Reagan's life.

T + 11 minutes after shooting: Reagan arrived at GWH and was allowed to walk into the Emergency room (ER), where he promptly collapsed. He should have been placed on a stretcher. Parr had called ahead for a stretcher which the hospital failed to provide. This was about the only mistake made by the hospital. President Reagan was then carried into the ER. He had no obtainable blood pressure at first measurement.

Dr. Joseph Giordano, chief of emergency services, said Reagan was close to death and that Agent Parr's decision to go directly to the hospital had saved the day. Dr. Giordano had organized the hospital's emergency response plan in 1979. It was the implementation of this plan that helped save Reagan's life.[5]

When Dr. Giordano arrived at the GWH Emergency Room, he was like a playwright watching the performance of his play (the emergency plan) by the actors (ER staff) that he had directed.

T + 11 to T +41 minutes post shooting: Within 30 minutes of arrival in the ER, Reagan had intravenous lines in place and saline infusions and blood transfusion had begun. An *endotracheal tube* was inserted, and CAT scans of the chest and abdomen were taken. He had *peritoneal* lavage, and a chest tube was inserted. The resident reneged on his promise to the student and did not let him insert Reagan's chest tube. Blood pressure was rapidly restored to normal, preoperatively. *Thoracic* surgery consultation was obtained, and routine preparation for chest surgery began.

T + 41 minutes post shooting: Reagan went to the OR and anesthesia and surgery were begun. The bullet was successfully removed from Reagan's chest. Postoperative care was uneventful.

. . .

CONSIDER the speed of delivery of care at this moment, only forty-one minutes from the moment of being shot. Compare Reagan's care with the slow-motion delivery of care for McKinley. Forty-one minutes after he was shot, McKinley was still waiting for the first doctor to arrive on the scene at the World Exposition.

Remember that the electric ambulance could have taken McKinley to Buffalo General Hospital in about fifteen minutes. The increased speed of Reagan's care had not been due to any technical innovation, but instead was due to having a plan based upon a premium of speed, of no waiting, of rapidly taking the patient to the place of definitive therapy.

This plan can be traced back to 1863, when wagoners at Gettysburg became dedicated ambulance drivers. Just before going into the OR, Reagan asked Dr. Giordano if all the doctors were Republicans. Chest surgeon Dr. Benjamin Aronson enjoyed telling Reagan (postop) that he was a lifelong Democrat.

THE CRITICAL MOMENTS were the 41 minutes from the shooting until entering OR.

From the shooting to ER: 11 minutes.

From the ER to the OR: 30 minutes.

Total: 41 minutes.

This is outstanding, excellent care, well within the time limits of the Golden Hour. Reagan's chest was explored, bleeding vessels tied off, and the bullet removed. Reagan made a rapid and complete recovery and returned to work.

This was a triumphant moment for American medicine. This was a team effort, and Giordano's emergency system was the star. It was the speed of the delivery of care that made the difference.

There was no need for a cover-up, no medical incompetence, no disability. The postoperative photos of Reagan in his bathrobe were a tonic for the nation.

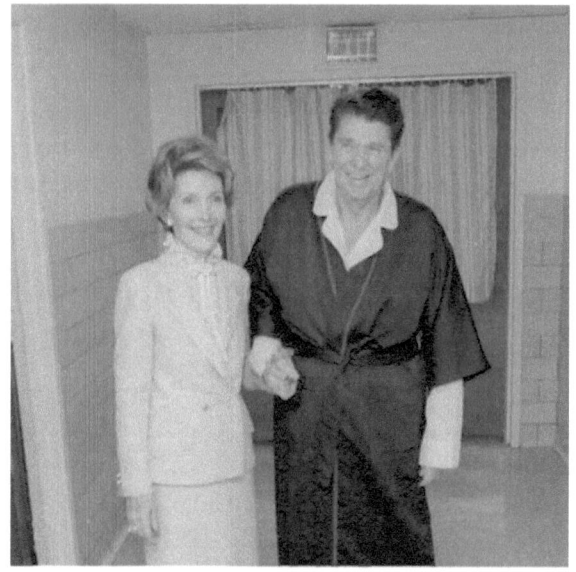

Image 17: The Reagans taking a post-operative stroll down hospital corridors at George Washington University, 1981

ONE HUNDRED YEARS separated the Garfield and Reagan shootings. Garfield should have survived his 1881 wound and almost certainly would have survived in 1981. Reagan would have probably died if he was shot in 1881, as there was not much thoracic surgery available.

In contrast to the outstanding medical care, and the bravery and skill of the Secret Service, the FBI put on a pitiful performance.

The FBI had told the doctors that Reagan was shot with a .38 caliber bullet. That statement was incorrect. The bullet seen on the chest X-ray was much smaller than a .38, so the doctors concluded that the bullet had fragmented. They used up precious time with a *peritoneal lavage* and abdominal *CAT* scan, looking for other fragments of the purported .38 caliber bullet. It was all unnecessary and a waste of precious time, because Reagan had not been shot with a .38 caliber bullet. In fact, he was shot with a .22 caliber bullet which had ricocheted off the car door and entered his chest. This was compatible with the bullet seen on the chest X-ray. There had been no need to look for any fragments.

Let's complete the evaluation of the response of the major players. The George Washington Hospital staff and the Secret Service knew what to do and did it well. The FBI provided erroneous and time-consuming information. The White House staff were not sure who was in charge while President Reagan was in surgery.

Let's also note Secretary of State Alexander Haig's famous comment after the shooting: "As of now, I am in control here, in the White House, pending the return of Vice President Bush." Haig would have been correct prior to 1947, but his comments in 1981 were contrary to the Presidential Succession Act of 1947 [6] which states that the line of succession was: President Reagan, VP Bush, Speaker of the House "Tip" O'Neill, the President Pro Tempore of the Senate, and then Secretary of State Al Haig and other following cabinet members.

The Presidential Succession Act of 1947 was the law of the land in 1981 and is still the law today. While Reagan was in surgery, VP George W. H. Bush was in Air Force 2 flying over Texas. Radio connections were poor, and Bush was only notified by secure teletype. He turned around and started flying back to Washington.[7]

In 1981, the speaker of the house was next in line of succession after the vice president. But Bush was alive and most observers believe that Bush automatically became acting president under Article 1, and/or Article 3 of the 25th Amendment. Upon reaching the hospital, Reagan was in shock and in no condition to activate Section 3 of the 25th Amendment with written declarations to the speaker of the house and the senate pro tempore.

The speaker could substitute for Bush only in an immediate emergency in the next hour or so until Bush landed and took charge. So, in fact Haig was fourth in line after VP Bush and Speaker Tip O'Neil and Senate President Pro Tempore Strom Thurmond.

Haig had got it very wrong and was 34 years behind the times. Haig's comment was also contrary to Reagan's plan for crisis management. That really annoyed other White House staff members present at the crisis. This incorrect declaration helped kill his career and in July 1982 he resigned as secretary of state.

Jim Baker stated that the 25th Amendment did not apply to Reagan's shooting, and no one challenged him. However, the amendment had been created to specifically deal with situations like Reagan's shooting. Baker got it wrong, except his comments were not televised to the nation as were Haig's.

ON JULY 13, 1985, Reagan underwent surgery at Bethesda Naval Hospital to remove cancerous polyps from his colon. He relinquished presidential power to the vice president for eight hours, following the guidelines in the 25th Amendment. Reagan specifically avoided invoking the 25th for uncertain reasons. The surgery lasted just under three hours and was successful.

President George W. Bush invoked the 25th Amendment on June 29, 2002, immediately before undergoing a colonoscopy, installing Vice President Dick Cheney as acting president. He was the first president to specifically cite Section 3 of the 25th Amendment in his letter temporarily transferring his powers and duties. President Bush repeated the whole process in July

2007. He earns a big plus for his place in history for these two peaceful legal transfers of power.

In 2021, it became apparent just how critical is the peaceful transfer of power. Because of these two peaceful transfers and his creation of the pandemic response office, George W. Bush clearly ranks above the quintet of Pierce, Buchanan, Johnson, Wilson, and Trump.

Bush's ranking as president is noted because the creation of the pandemic office and the implementation of the 25th amendment are all about health care. His actions were critical for the health and security of the nation.

Finally, did Ronald Reagan have Alzheimer's disease when he was President? He was the second oldest man ever to be president. He took afternoon naps and was forgetful at times. This, however, is insufficient evidence for a diagnosis of Alzheimer's disease.

Reagan left office in January 1989. That July, he was thrown from a horse, suffering head trauma and a subdural hematoma that was surgically treated two months later. A comprehensive neurological evaluation at that time showed no signs of dementia.

In 1991, he appeared on the Larry King Show to answer questions about the 1981 shooting. His memory, intellect and speech were intact, and he did not appear to have Alzheimer's disease.[8]

In August 1994, at the age of 83, Reagan was diagnosed with Alzheimer's disease, five years after leaving the presidency. In June 2004, President Ronald Reagan died at the age of 93. He had suffered from Alzheimer's for 10 years, from 1994 to 2004. This was significantly longer than the average duration of 4 to 8 years. To imply that he had Alzheimer's during his presidency would stretch the duration of his disease for a total of 23 years (1981-2004). Did Reagan Alzheimer's begin during his presidency? Probably not. Allegations are neither evidence nor proof, not in medical diagnoses and not in disputed election results.

Final notes on this topic from an article published in the *New York Times* by the authoritative Dr. Lawrence Altman, MD. "As a follow-up to questions about Alzheimer's, my extensive interviews with his White House doctors, key aides and others, I found no evidence that Mr. Reagan exhibited signs of dementia. Our interviews did not include family members." [9]

EPILOGUE

In 2021, Joe Biden became President, the 46th man holding the office. At 80 years old, he is the oldest president ever but appears to be in good health. His speech impediments are not the sign of any neurological disease but are manifestations of his lifelong stammer and stutter.

Biden supports modern science, condemns xenophobia, and places independent distinguished scientists at leadership positions at CDC and FDA, and as surgeon general. His administration proposed a multi-billion-dollar pandemic preparedness program. He always wears a mask in public and supports those who also do that. He comes out strongly against the medical quackery still prevalent in the land. The US has rejoined the world, specifically the World Health Organization.

According to the *Wall Street Journal*, we live in the golden age of "monumental stupidity," where basic science appears unknown, and President Biden has a tough job to keep it altogether.

On January 6, 2021, an insurrection in Washington, DC tried to stop the completion of the electoral vote. It was broadcast live on TV and widely viewed. Yet millions of Americans believe it never happened. How do you respond to this? As the old joke goes "who do you believe, me or your lying eyes?"

The country is divided into two camps: anti-science versus pro-science. The split has been present since someone firebombed Dr. Boylston's home in 1721 because he inoculated people against smallpox. The nation is divided today as at no time since the Civil War of 1861.

There are four issues to consider how we arrived at this contentious moment in history.

The first is to consider our obsolete electoral process for the presidency. As mentioned earlier, the peaceful transition of power has been threatened several times. The 25th Amendment provides some progress but removing a disabled president against his will appears to be unlikely.

Are we to repeat the disgrace of Edith Wilson as acting president?

In the case of electoral voting disputes, the 12th Amendment left us with the partisan involvement of the House of Representatives, with each state having one vote. How nondemocratic is that?

Finally, the electoral college, with separate state votes, audits, and recording of votes is anathema for a democracy. The involvement of the state legislatures is contrary to the concept of a national election. The electoral college needs to go into the dustbin of history. It has no place in a modern democracy.

THE SECOND ISSUE is the rise and fall of public health. That has been closely linked with the public benefits of implementation of the germ theory of infectious diseases. By 1910, the tipping point had been achieved, as the public benefited by having vaccines for smallpox and rabies, antitoxins for diphtheria and tetanus, and filtered drinking water to prevent cholera. The progress continued with the development of a safe and effective Yellow Fever vaccine in 1937.

The highlight was the development by Jonas Salk of the polio vaccine in 1955. His research was supported by the March of Dimes, which was organized by FDR. Public financial support of the research led to powerful support for vaccination, and the involvement of FDR was a master stroke of public relations. The public felt connected to FDR and understood the concept of the March of Dimes. In addition, FDR's charisma and political skills overwhelmed any opposition to vaccinations.

But support for public health has evaporated in recent years. Health departments have been decimated as public spending for public health declined. Almost no public health is taught in public school and there are far fewer school nurses than ever before.

There is a great need to reinvent public health education in the US and to restore public health services to a more robust status. To do that might require amending state constitutions to remove governors and legislatures from interfering in public health emergencies.

There exists another divide between the entitled and the common folk. Recall that Mary Montagu, a friend of the Queen of England, persuaded the elite of England to get inoculated against smallpox. The aristocracy, the royals, the university educated, and the Army were inoculated, the rest of England to a lesser degree. In America, with no aristocracy, there was less advocacy for inoculation.

A different set of rules seem to exist for celebrities. Jackie Kennedy broke the law and prevented JFK's autopsy being done in Dallas, which led to 58 years of nonstop controversy. Stanford University Hospital executives got COVID vaccinations days before frontline health care workers. Hollywood actress Nicole Kidman avoided quarantine at Hong Kong Airport. Private citizen Bill Clinton boarded an airplane on the tarmac to speak with the US attorney general. Mickey Mantle, Steve Jobs, and Governor Robert Casey of Pennsylvania may have used their wealth and/or celebrity to jump the queue of the organ transplant system.

THE THIRD ISSUE is the public distrust of government. Examples are Watergate, Vietnam, the Gulf of Tonkin Resolution, JFK's assassination, 9/11 and the incompetence of the FBI and CIA, the futile search for weapons of mass destruction in Iraq, the 20-year US involvement in Afghanistan. This leads many to believe that government cannot be trusted. That lack of trust extends to questions about vaccines, the ingredients in the vaccine, and morphs into the larger question of vaccine safety. Why place faith in Big Pharma that in recent years has been making huge profits from the exorbitant prices they charge?

The cover-ups in the 19th century were almost comical, but in the 20th century they have had dire consequences. The price paid for the Wilson cover-up was Red Raids in the US, a punitive armistice for Germany, and a weakened peace treaty and League of Nations. The price FDR paid for the cover-up of his heart failure was his disastrous trip to Yalta. For JFK, the cover-up of his medical history and drug use led to his use of amphetamines during the Cuban Missile Crisis.

THE FOURTH ISSUE, incompetent medical care for the president. The White House physician needs to be a well-qualified physician who performs as a civil servant with no encumbering military chain of command. The White House physician could be supported and reviewed by an independent medical review body appointed by an independent group, like the National Science Foundation. The primary loyalty of the White House physician has to be the president, but they cannot lie or obfuscate with their public pronouncements. They need to have the prestige and authority to protect the president. They need to step up to the plate and say, "President Roosevelt, you are not well enough to travel to Yalta."

What if a madman became president and threatened to blow up the world? It might be more practical to place safeguards in the nuclear chain of command than to screen presidential candidates for incipient mental disease.

It is the potential for repeated cover-ups of presidential disease that remains so troublesome. How much privacy do you give up when you run for president? I propose that you have to give up a lot, and I would leave the details to the independent review board that will be created.

WE BEGAN the American phase of our narrative with attempts to control the 1721 smallpox epidemic. We are still coping with a national outbreak of Covid 19 due to the failure of public health policy. In 1721, opponents of smallpox vaccine firebombed Dr. Boylston's home. In 2020, opponents of Covid 19 quarantines tried to murder Governor Whitmer of Michigan. This is not progress.

A tip of the hat to our unsung heroes: Onesimus, Cotton Mather, Mary Montagu, Zebdiel Boylston, John Riker, Anna Roosevelt and Howard Bruenn, Bette Jackson and the thousands of women of the Continental Army, Ignace Semmelweis, Walt Whitman, Ephraim McDowell, William Beaumont, Crawford Long, Oliver Wendell Holmes Sr., William Halstead, William Gorgas, Charles Drew, Dwight Harkens, Thomas Mattingly, Rene Favaloro, Jerry Parr, Charles Giordano, and to Florence Nightingale and all the great nurses who bring the caring to medical care.

As of March 2021, there have been 3,700 health care workers who have died on the front lines of the Covid 19 wars. A grateful nation remembers them with undying support and love.

. . .

For a final thought, let's remember another moment in history when the nation was torn in two and the 600,000 Americans who died during the Civil War. We don't have another Lincoln, but we have his words, and that should be enough.

"With malice toward none; with charity for all; with firmness in the right, as God gives us to see the right, let us strive on to finish the work we are in; to bind up the nation's wounds; to care for him who shall have borne the battle, and for his widow, and his orphan—to do all which may achieve and cherish a just, and a lasting peace, among ourselves, and with all nations."

ENDNOTES

Introduction

1. *Lyndon Johnson and Franklin Delano Roosevelt (FDR) also made major contributions to medical care. Lyndon Johnson was the chief advocate for the Medicare Act of 1965, which brought medical care to millions. FDR was the moving force behind the March of Dimes which culminated in the polio vaccines developed by Dr. Salk and Dr. Sabin. ELG*

2. *Neither Wilson nor Trump recognized the dire consequences of pandemics and failed to act appropriately. ELG*

3. Chen, C. (2003). "On the Shoulders of Giants." In *Mapping Scientific Frontiers:* The Quest for Knowledge Visualization. Springer, London. 1978

4. *Appropriate starting point for the text are the Boston riots of 1721 that were in response to smallpox inoculation. ELG*

5. *I first heard of this concept from Dr Franz Ingelfinger, erstwhile editor of the New England Journal Medicine in a public lecture in Boston, circa 1978. ELG*

6. Duffy, Thomas P. MD, "The Flexner Report 100 Years Later," *Yale Journal of Biology and Medicine* 2011 Sep; 84(3): 269–276. Published online September 2011

7. Rich, Frank, "Has He Started Talking to the Walls?", *New York Times,* December 3, 2006.

"It turns out we have been reading the wrong Bob Woodward book to understand what's going on with President Bush. The text we should be consulting instead is *The Final Days,* the Woodward-Bernstein account of Richard Nixon talking to the portraits on the White House walls while Watergate demolished his presidency.

Chapter 1 A. Smallpox

1. "History of Smallpox." https://*www.cdc.gov smallpox history,* February 20, 2021

Discussion of smallpox disease is mainly from CDC Bulletins. ELG.

2. Choi, Charles Q "Case Closed? Columbus Introduced Syphilis to Europe," *Scientific American,* December 27, 2011.

Syphilis apparently had been present in the New World for thousands of years. That theory is supported by examining the skeletal remains of North American women found at archeological sites. Many of the skeletons have bone lesions suggestive of syphilis. Radioactive dating of these skeletons shows these lesions were present thousands of years before Columbus. But this remains an unsettled scientific issue. ELG

3. Tampa, I Sarbu, SR Georgescu, SR, "Brief History of Syphilis", *Journal of Medicine and Life,* March 14, 2014, page 5.

4.tp://www.webster.edu/~corbetre/haiti/history/pre-columbian/tainover.htm

5. Prine Pauls, Elizabeth "Native American." *Encyclopedia Britannica,* 17 Aug. 2021, Accessed 6 November 2021.

6. Chernow, Ron, *Grant,* Penguin Press, New York, pp 658-9.

7. d'Errico, Peter *Daily Hampshire, Letters,*8/19/2, "Jeffery Amherst and Smallpox Blankets."

8. "Smallpox the Threat" *CDC,* Page last reviewed: December 19, 2016.

Philadelphia —Nov 18, 2021 CBS news. Federal health authori-

ties on Wednesday confirmed the discovery of some frozen vials labeled "Smallpox" in a freezer at a facility in Pennsylvania that conducts vaccine research. The Centers for Disease Control and Prevention said the vials "were incidentally discovered by a laboratory worker" who was cleaning out the freezer. CDC, its administration partners, and law enforcement are investigating the matter and the vials' contents appear intact," CDC spokesperson Belsie González said in an email.

9. "Smallpox, Signs and Symptoms," *CDC*, Last reviewed June 7, 2016

10. Adi, Hakim, *BBC History*, "Africa and the Transatlantic Slave Trade," Last updated 2012-10-05.

11. Augustan, Adam, editor, "Middle Passage Slave Ship" *Encyclopedia Britannica*.

12. Dauril, Alden and Joseph C. Miller. "Out of Africa: The Slave Trade and the "Transmission of Smallpox to Brazil," 1560-1831." *The Journal of Interdisciplinary History,* vol. 18, no. 2, The MIT Press, 1987, pp. 195–224.

13. Reidel, Stefan, MD. PhD. "Edward Jenner and the History of Smallpox and Vaccines," *Baylor University Medical Center Proceedings,* vol 18, 2005

14. Neiderhuber, Matthew, *Special Edition Infectious Disease.* "Science in the News, Harvard University." December 31, 2014.

15 Beal Jr, O.T., *Bulletin History Medicine,*

16. Fries, Gwen "Living in an Epidemic: What Did Abigail Do?" *The Beehive*, official blog of the Massachusetts Historical Society, April 30, 2020. https://www.masshist.org/beehiveblog/2020/05/living-in-an-epidemic-what-did-abigail-do/

Abigail Adams kept herself informed, was proactive, and monitored her physical health during the two months that she and the children were isolated with smallpox.

17. Witt, John Fabian, *New York Times, October 16, 2020.* "Gibbons v Ogden: Opinion." Republican judges overturning public health laws.

Chapter 1 B. Smallpox and the American Revolution

1. Fenn, Elizabeth, *Pox Americana*, New York, Hill and Wang, 2001 *This book provided much of the factual narrative for the seven-year North American epidemic of smallpox 1775-1782. ELG*

2. "Retreat from Quebec" *Journal of Military History*, Vol. 68, No. 2 (Apr 2004).

3. Atkinson, Rick, *The British are Coming*, New York, Henry Holt and Co., P 84-139, pp 220-240, 257-271.

This was my major source of information for the siege of Boston. Also of note was Fischer, David Hackett, Washington's Crossing, Oxford University Press, USA. page 9, That was about the Loyalists leaving Boston. ELG

4. Atkinson, p 235

5. *Only the heroic stand of the 1st Maryland Regiment allowed the bulk of the Continental troops to avoid capture and retire safely to Brooklyn Heights on Long Island. Under the cover of fog, the Continental Army miraculously escaped from Long Island. Every manner of boat was used: canoes, rowboats, sloops, sailboats, and barges to cross the East River from Brooklyn Heights to Manhattan. More than 9,000 Continental troops were evacuated with no further loss of life, Washington being the last man to leave. ELG*

6. *The Crisis*, Thomas Paine, History.com editors. Original Published December 19,1776

7. Bumgarner, John, R, MD, *The Health of the Presidents*, McFarland and Co., Jefferson, North Carolina, p32.

This book was my major source of biographical information for the presidents. ELG

8. Gianakon, Julie, "Doctor Riker's Decision," Philadelphia, *Hektoen International: A Journal of Medical Humanities.* January 2017

9. Geppert, Cynthia M.A., MD and Paul, Reid A., "The Shot that Won the Revolutionary War and Is Still Reverberating," *Federal Practitioner*, July 2019

10. Fenn, ibid; "George Washington's Trip to Barbados."

11. Watkins, Jack, "Journey to Barbados," Mt Vernon Organi-

zation.https://www.mountvernon.org/george-washington/washingtons-youth/journey-to-barbados/

12. "*Sullivan's Campaign. The Clinton-Sullivan Campaign of 1779,*" compiled by Fort Stanwix Staff, Fort Stanwix, NY, National Park Service.

As the British were losing allies, (Loyalists and Iroquois) about 100 professional soldiers and foreign mercenaries joined the Continental Army and made outstanding contributions. They include Johan De Kalb, Baron von Steuben, Casimir Pulaski, Tadeusz Kosciusko, the Marquis de Lafayette, and Moses Hazen (Canadian-American). With the entry of French army and navy in the war in 1778, actual victory for the Continentals became possible. ELG

13. Buchanan, John, "*The Road to Charleston: Nathanael Greene and the American Revolution,*" Charlottesville, University of Virginia Press, 2019.

Nathanael Greene's brilliant 1781 campaign in the Carolinas relied upon the basic tactic of keeping a river, stream, swamp, or some obstacle between his forces and his pursuer, General Cornwallis, commander of British forces in the South. The race to the Dan River was a classic example of this, as Greene managed to keep Cornwallis on the run. This was an example of classic Fabian strategy. Avoid large, fixed battles, and keep the army intact and always on the move. ELG

14. William S. Powell, "Seasoning Period," *Encyclopedia of North Carolina,* 2006.

15. In 1780 during the siege of Charleston, South Carolina, thousands of local militiamen who were not smallpox immune refused to enter and defend the city because Charleston was in the midst of a smallpox epidemic. That led to the worst Continental defeat of the Revolutionary War, as 5,000 Continental troops within the city surrendered to the British.

16. Whitman, Walt, "The Wallabout Martyrs," *Leaves of Grass,* Brooklyn, NY, 1855–1892, self-published, Brooklyn Eagle, 1888.

17. Bumgarner ibid, p 43-44

18. Remini, Robert, *The Life of Andrew Jackson,* Penguin New York 1990, p9

Chapter 2. Frontier Medicine

1. Parascandola, J., "Drug Therapy in Colonial and Revolutionary America," *American Journal of Hospital Pharmacology,* August 1976, vol 33, pp. 807-810

2. "Medicine," *Liberty! Chronicle of the Revolution.* PBS.org, 2004.https://www.pbs.org/ktca/liberty/chronicle_subject.html

3. Sarudy, Barbara Wells, "Lucy Meriwether Lewis," *Women in 19C America,* https://b-womeninamericanhistory19.blogspot.com/2019/05/lucy-meriwether-lewis-marks1752-1837.html, May 24, 2019.

4. Jones, Randell, "Westward Expansion," *Smoky Mountain Living,* April 1, 2019

5. Roosevelt, Theodore, *Winning the West,* Simon and Schuster, 1889, 2021, Chapter V, "The Backwoodsman of the Alleghenies." Chapter X, "Boone and the Settlement of Kentucky."

6. Othersen, Jr., H Biemann MD, "Ephraim McDowell: Qualities of a Good Surgeon," *Annals of Surgery,* 2004 May; 239(5): 648–650.

7. "William Beaumont" *Encyclopedia Britannica,* 12 Nov. 2021.

8. Anaya-Prado R, Schadegg-Peña D. "Crawford Williamson Long: The True Pioneer of Surgical Anesthesia," *J Investigational Surgery.* 2015;28(4):181-7.

9. Strauss, Maurice B, "Sir Francis Darwin and Sir William Osler," *J American Medical Association,* 1966;196 (31):1161. "In science, credit goes to the man who convinces the world, not the man to whom the idea first occurs." Crawford Long v William Morton" Quote is from Francis Darwin

10. Mays, Jeffrey C. and Small, Zachary "Thomas Jefferson Statue Evicted from New York City Hall, Will Go to a Museum," *New York Times,* November 15, 2021.

Heeding requests to move Jefferson's statue because of his legacy as an enslaver, New York City approved a plan to relocate it to the

New York Historical Society. One wonders if those in charge knew of the Northwest Ordinance of 1785. ELG

Chapter 3. Long Guns

1. "Daniel Boone escorting settlers through the Cumberland Gap". George Caleb Bingham, artist. Washington University Gallery of Art, St. Louis, Mo, US, 1852.

2. *"The Man Who Shot Liberty Valance" is a 1962 American western film directed by John Ford that starred John Wayne and James Stewart. The film was selected for the 1962 States Registry by the Library of Congress as being "culturally, historically, or aesthetically significant." The famous line from the movie is "This is the West, sir. When the legend becomes fact, print the legend." ELG*

3. Bumgarner, p117.

4. Bumgarner, p119.

5. O'Toole, Patricia, "The Speech That Saved Teddy Roosevelt's Life," *Smithsonian Magazine*, November 2012.

6. Smith, ibid *FDR* p 297

7. *This is an apocryphal quote, yet it is inscribed on Cermak's tomb. There has never been any specific attribution. ELG*

8. December 17, 1975, HISTORY TV, Lynette "Squeaky" Fromme sentenced to life for assassination attempt. Articles with the "HISTORY.com Editors" byline have been written or edited by HISTORY editors, including Amanda Onion, Missy Sullivan and Matt Mulle.

9. Rangel, Jesus "Obituary Oliver W. Sipple, 47, who Blocked an Attempt To Kill Ford in 1975." February 4, 1989, *New York Times*.

10. UPI Archives April 13, 1981. The president of the Jewish Carpenters Local 1750 was Alfred Antenucci, an Italian Catholic. Antenucci, then 68, was standing close to John Hinckley as he attempted to assassinate President Ronald Reagan. He struck Hinckley and took him to the ground, spoiling his aim.

Chapter 4. Louisiana

1. McCutcheon, Jennifer Monroe, "Proclamation Line 1763," *George Washington's Mount Vernon Organization, Texas Christian University*, c/o 2022, Mt. Vernon Ladies' Association.

2. Treaty of Paris 1783, US Dept. State Archive.

3. "Traveler's Health", *CDC*, 2021.

4. "Life Cycle Aedes Mosquito," *CDC,* March 5, 2020.

5. Cathey, J.T. Marr J.S. "Yellow Fever in Africa and the Americas: An Historical and Epidemiological Perspective. *Trans Royal Society of Tropical Medicine and Hygiene.* 2014, May, 108 (5): 252-7.

6. Opal, JM and Opal, Steven, "When Mosquitos Brought Yellow Fever to the Caribbean, They Also Brought Slavery," *TIME,* October 11, 2019.

7. Gum, Samuel A, "Philadelphia Under Siege: The Yellow Fever of 1793," Pennsylvania Center for the Book. https://web.archive.org/web/20220804001159/https://pabook.libraries.psu.edu/literary-cultural-heritage-map-pa/feature-articles/philadelphia-under-siege-yellow-fever-1793

8. These letters are part of the Wyck Association Collection, which was recently donated to the American Philosophical Society (APS).

9. *For a more detailed account, of the Louisiana Purchase, I recommend Henry Adams' History of the United States of America during the Administrations of Thomas Jefferson (1801–1809), especially pages 269 to 545. You may explore further the exact role of the Baring's Bank, which already had significant dealings in the US, but that is a topic for another book. In 1995, the bank collapsed following fraudulent investments of $1.7 billion by one employee at their Singapore office. Baring's had been in business since 1762. ELG*

10. *Benjamin Franklin, the first president of the American Philosophical Society, was also a member of the British Royal Society. He was probably the premier scientist in the New World in first half of eighteenth century. He had many scientific inventions and accomplishments.*

Franklin was one of the founders of the University of Pennsylvania in 1740, and that is now the fifth oldest university in the nation. Its medical school is the oldest in United States, founded in 1765. Franklin was also one of the founders of the University of Pennsylvania Hospital in 1751, the oldest continuously functioning hospital in the US.

Franklin invented bifocal eyeglasses, discovered and mapped the Gulf Stream. He discovered the concept of positive and electrical charges of electricity, the lightning rod, along with the concept that lightning is an electric charge. It is extraordinary that two of our nation's founding parents were first-rate scientists. Franklin and Jefferson gave a fantastic gift to the new republic, their love of science, which soon became an indelible part of American culture. ELG

11. Roosevelt, Theodore, *Winning the West*, Simon and Schuster, 1889, 2021, Daniel Boone at the Yellowstone River.

12. Kennedy, John F. "Remarks at a Dinner Honoring Nobel Prize Winners of the Western Hemisphere," 29 April. 1962. Published by Gerhard Peters and John T. Woolley, editors,

American Presidency Project (accessed 2014). *Jefferson is part of another long thread, the study of the natural world. That same thread stretches back to the ancient Greeks, and is also attached to Jenner to Lister, to Pasteur, to Gorgas, to Salk and others. This thread continues to the present day. ELG*

13. "Yellow Fever: The plague of Memphis." Historic Memphis. http://www.historic-memphis.com/memphis-historic/yellow-fever/yellow-fever.html.

14. Weisberger, Bernard A. "Memphis Fights the Yellow Fever." *American Heritage, October-November 1984*

A disease that no one understood laid waste a major American city as five thousand people died in two months. Most white residents died, and most black residents survived. There is no explanation for this racial disparity. ELG

Chapter 5. Great Men, Great Women, Great Ideas

1. Rhodes, Philip; Guthrie, Douglas James; Richardson, Robert G.; Thomson, William, Robson, Archibald, and Underwood; E Ashworth. "History of Medicine, 18th–19th century" *Encyclopedia Britannica*, 27 August 2020, P. 71

2. *Changes in Health and Medicine, 1340 to present*, BBC, P 72

3. Ibid.

4. Fitzharris, Lindsey. "One Night with Venus, a Lifetime with Mercury: Syphilis and Syphilophobes in Early Modern England." The Chirugeon's Apprentice, December 22, 2010. https://drlindseyfitzharris.com/one-night-with-venus-a-lifetime-with-mercury-syphilis-and-syphilophobes-in-early-modern-england/

5. Riedel, Stefan MD PhD. "Edward Jenner and the History of Smallpox and Vaccination"*Proceedings,* Baylor University Medical Center, 2005, Jan 18 (1): pp21-25

"In science, credit goes to the man who convinces the world, not the man to whom the idea first occurs". Credited to Francis Darwin, the son of Charles Darwin.

6. Morabia, Alfredo. "Pierre-Charles-Alexandre-Louis and the Evaluation of Bloodletting," *Journal Royal Society London*, 2006 Mar; 99 (3): pp 230-235.

7. Rogers, Kara and Rougin, Ariel. "Biography Rene Laennec" *Encyclopedia Britannica*

8. Rougin, Ariel MD, PhD, "Rene Theophile Hyacinthe Laennec (1781-1826) The Man Behind the Stethoscope, *Clinical Medical Research*, 2006, Septemeber; 4(3): pp 230-235.

9. "Joseph Skoda (1805-1881) Physical Diagnostician," Editorial, *JAMA*, October 19,1964; p 240

10. Sakula, A. "Joseph Skoda 1805-1881: a Centenary Tribute to a Pioneer of Thoracic Medicine" *Thorax* 1981;36(6): pp 404-411

11. Editors of Encyclopedia Britannica. "Oliver Wendell Holmes. Encyclopedia Britannica, October 3, 2022. https://www.britannica.com/biography/Oliver-Wendell-Holmes

12. Holmes, Oliver Wendell, statement made at Massachusetts Medical Society, May 1860.

"Currents and Counter currents in Modern Medicine," *The American Journal of Medicine 1860* Paraphrased version: "If all the medicine in the world were thrown into the sea, it would be bad for the fish and good for humanity."

13. Nuland, Sherwin B. *The Doctor's Plague: Germs, Childbed fever and the Strange Story of Ignacio Semmelweis,* Norton/Alas Books, 2003

14. Vertanen, Reino, "Claude Bernard." *Encyclopedia Britannica,* July 2021. https://www.britannica.com/biography/Claude-Bernard

15. Schultz, Myron: "Rudolph Virchow." *Emerging Infectious Diseases,* 2008, pp 1480-1481.

16. Mitali, Banerjee Ruths, MD, "The Lesson of John Snow and the Broad Street Pump, "*Virtual Mentor,* 2009

17. Fitzharris, Lindsey, "The Butchering Art." New York, *Scientific American*, 2017, p149-160

18. Ibid., p.169

19. Ibid., p.169

20. Ibid., p. 207

21. Ibid., p. 215

22. Cartwright, Frederick F.,"Joseph Lister" *Encyclopedia Britannica*, June 2021, https://www.britannica.com/biography/Joseph-Lister-Baron-Lister-of-Lyme-Regis.

23. Ullman, Agnes, "Louis Pasteur" *Encyclopedia Britannica*, December 2021. https://www.britannica.com/biography/Louis-Pasteur.

24. Smith, K.A. "Louis Pasteur, The Father of Immunology." *Frontier Immunology,* April, 2012.

25. Ibid Smith, In 1798 Jenner wrote, "Inquiry into the the Variolae Vaccinae, Known as the Cow Pox," in which he described the protective effects of cowpox against smallpox. That process is called vaccination.

That change would go on to confuse generations of medical

students who struggled with the concept that smallpox vaccine was not derived from smallpox virus. The term vaccine is now used to describe any preparation of weakened or killed bacteria or viruses introduced in the body to prevent a disease, by stimulating antibodies directed against it. That brings us to the Covid Vaccine. ELG

26. Robert Koch-Biographical. Nobel Prize.org. Nobel Prize Outreach AB 2022 https://www.nobelprize.org/prizes/medicine/1905/koch/biographical

27. Segre, Julia, "Koch's Postulates." *Journal of Investigative Dermatology*, 2013, pp 2141-2

28. Segre, Ibid.

29. Burns, Ken, "The Roosevelts, Part 2:, In the Arena." PBS Television 2014.

30. "TR and the Panama Canal.",*American Experience*, PBS Television, 2011.

31. Ibid.

32. Ibid.

33. Ibid.

34. Ibid.

35. "Yellow Fever Virus," Center for Disease Control and Prevention, April 21, 2022, https://www.cdc.gov/yellowfever/index.html

Chapter 6. Transfer of Power

1. White, Adam"A Republic If you Can Keep It." *The Atlantic*, February 4, 2020

2. Bumgarner, John, *The Health of the Presidents* McFarland and Co. Jefferson North Carolina and London, 1994 p1-301

3. Bumgarner Ibid. p 29.

4. National Archives. Devolve Clause. US Constitution.

5. *End note Disputed elections have sorely tested the peaceful transfer of power. ELG*

1800. Thirty-five ballots in the House of Representatives required to elect Jefferson, leading to the passage of the 12th

Amendment that simplified the electoral process, and mandated separate ballots forPresident and vice president.

1824. Jackson vs John Quincy Adams vs Henry Clay vs William Crawford. No candidate received a majority of the electoral college vote, so the president was selected by the House of Representatives. Henry Clay, the Speaker of the House, threw his support behind John Quincy Adams and that gave him the election. In return Quincy Adams nominated Clay to be secretary of state. Andrew Jackson and friends responded by forming the national Democratic Party.

1860. Lincoln vs Douglas vs Bell vs Breckinridge. Lincoln did win the majority of the electoral college votes, but his victory led to the secession of the South and the subsequent Civil War.

1876. Hayes vs Tilden. There were problems counting the vote in Southern states occupied by federal troops. The election was a travesty. Samuel Tilden had won the popular vote by 260,000 votes but was shy one electoral vote. Nineteen electoral votes from Florida, South Carolina, and Louisiana were in dispute.

A partisan electoral commission made a Corrupt Bargain. They gave all those disputed votes to Hayes, who was then elected president. In return federal troops withdrew from the South and Black Americans were no longer protected by the federal government. Jim Crow laws prevailed for the next eighty-eight years. The presidential parade now had a stink about it that lasted until the Civil Rights Acts of 1964-1965.

2000. Gore vs Bush. Hanging chads in Florida required the intervention of the U.S. Supreme Court to decide the election in favor of Bush

2020. Trump vs Biden. A mob of Trump supporters stormed the US Capitol on January 6, 2021 trying to stop the counting of the Electoral College vote and overturn 224 years of non-violent transition of power.

Chapter 7. Parade of Presidents

1. Widmer, Ted. "Draining the Swamp."*The New Yorker*, January 19, 2017. From the beginning, the creators of Washington, DC went to some trouble to conceal that their capital was a swamp.

2. "History of the Cherry Trees," Cherry Blossom Festival NPS.gov. https://www.nps.gov/subjects/cherryblossom/history-of-the-cherry-trees.htm

3. Hacker, J David. "Decennial Life Tables for the White Population of the United States, 1790-1900", *Historical Methods* vol 43,2 (2010): 45-79 doi:10.1080/01615441003720449.

4. "Adams Family Tree" *Massachusetts Historical Society.* https://www.masshist.org/adams/family-tree

The two Adams presidents and their descendants are descended from John Alden, and Priscilla Mullins, who came to the United States on the *Mayflower*. The Adams are one of four families to have produced two presidents of the United States, the others being the Bush, Roosevelt, and Harrison families. The following are the highlights of this extraordinary Adams family tree.

John Alden and Priscilla Mullins, passengers on the Mayflower, are great-great-great parents of John Adams.

Samuel Adams (1722–1803), revolutionary, delegate to the Continental Congress and governor of Massachusetts, was John Adams' second cousin.

John Adams, (1735–1826), second president of U.S., married to Abigail Adams (née Smith) (1744–1818).

John Quincy Adams (1767–1848), sixth president of the United States.

Charles Francis Adams. (1807-1886). US congressman and ambassador to the United Kingdom during US Civil War.

Henry Adams (1838–1918), prominent author and political commentator,

Brooks Adams (1848–1927), historian and political scientist.

(Henry and Brooks were brothers, and grandsons of John Quincy Adams and sons to Charles Francis Adams)

5. "Wrist Injury" The Thomas Jefferson Encyclopedia. *The Thomas Jefferson Monticello.* https://www.monticello.org/research-education/thomas-jefferson-encyclopedia/wrist-injury-1786/

6. Deppisch, L.M. "Andrew Jackson's Exposure to Mercury and Lead: A Poisoned President" *JAMA.* 1999 August 11;282(6):569-71 Brief Report

7. Bumgarner, pages 53-54, Amyloidosis is presented as being caused by bronchiectasis and/or heavy metal poisoning.

8. Martin Van Buren suffered from chronic gouty arthritis, which can be treated with the drug colchicine, introduced into the US by Benjamin Franklin.

9. "W.H.Harrison,"The FDA History Office. https://www.fda.gov/about-fda/fda-history/fda-history-office. *Harrison probably died from salmonella enteritis, a food borne disease. The original Food and Drugs Act was passed by Congress on June 30, 1906 and signed by President Theodore Roosevelt.*

It prohibits interstate commerce in misbranded and adulterated foods, drinks, and drugs. The Meat Inspection Act was passed the next day. Shocking disclosures, of unsanitary conditions in meat-packing plants, the use of poisonous preservatives and dyes in foods, and cure-all claims for worthless and dangerous patent medicines were the major problems leading to the enactment of these laws. They were the highlights of The Jungle written by Upton Sinclair. ELG

10. John Tyler, McFadden, Robert D. "Lyon Taylor, Dies at age 95," *New York Times,* October 7, 2020.

His brother Harrison, age 93 is the last remaining grandson of President John Tyler, who was born in 1790, only 232 years ago. John Tyler could be considered as "father of the country" with his fifteen children with his two wives. ELG

On February 28, 1844, President Tyler was in the company of Dolly Madison aboard the USS Princeton when a "Peacemaker"

cannon exploded. Secretary of State Abel P. Upshur and Secretary of Navy Thomas Walker Gilmer were killed, but President Tyler and Dolly Madison both escaped unharmed. This was another close call for the US, and the process of peaceful transition of power. If Tyler had been killed, the presidency would have passed to the President Pro-tempore of the Senate, an un-elected official. ELG

11. Goldman, Arnold S and Frank C. Schmalstieg, Jr. "Abraham Lincoln's Gettysburg Illness," Journal of Medical Biography vol 15,2 (2007) 104-10 doi:10.1258/j.jmb.2007.06-14

12. "Smallpox. Center for Disease Control and Prevention" https://www.cdc.gov/smallpox/index.html.

Last case of Smallpox in the US was in 1949.

13. Emerson, Jason "How Edwin Booth Save the Life of Robert Todd Lincoln" https://www.historynet.com/edwin-booth-saved-robert-todd-lincolns-life-2/

In an ironic twist of fate, Edwin Booth, the brother of John Wilkes Booth, Lincoln''s assassin, saved the life of the president's eldest son Robert in the winter of 1864. Both men had been standing on a train platform in Jersey City, New Jersey, when Robert Lincoln fell off the platform, alongside a moving train. Booth picked Lincoln up by the coat collar, bringing him safety back onto the platform. ELG

Jason Emerson originally published this in the April 2005 issue of Civil War Times. ELG

14. Yow AG, Rajasurya V, Sharma S. "TR Sudden death." Updated 2021 Aug 12 *StatPearls* [Internet]. Treasure Island (FL): StatPearls Publishing; 2022 Jan

15. "Exhume the Body of Warren G. Harding? A Judge Says That Won't Be Necessary" *New York Times,* December 1, 2020, https://www.nytimes.com/2020/12/01/us/warren-harding-grand son-exhume.html

16. Beatty, Jack. "Review: The Tormented President: Calvin Coolidge, Death and Clinical Depression," *Atlantic,* December 31, 2003, https://www.theatlantic.com/past/docs/unbound/polipro/pp2003-12-31.htm

This biography placed Coolidge's presidency in the context of the deep depression into which he fell following the death of his son. The Boston Globe wrote, "President Coolidge was more communicative than any previous President with the possible exception of Theodore Roosevelt." After his son's death, Coolidge earned the nickname "*Silent Cal*"

17. American Psychiatric Association

18. Hoover, Herbert, 1874-1964 Person Authority Record, archives.gov/ under-secretary of everything

19. *Principles of Medical Ethics: Section 7* American Psychiatric Association (APA). Original Publication: 1973 APA's Principles of Medical Ethics, states that " ...a psychiatrist may share with the public his or her expertise about psychiatric issues in general. However, it is unethical for a psychiatrist to offer a professional opinion unless he or she has conducted an examination and has been granted proper authorization for such a statement." This is the Goldwater Rule, which is still in effect

20. Altman, Lawrence K."Nixon's Leg Worsens." New York Times September 13, 1974

21. *There are multiple inconclusive reports re: who won the debates Nixon v JFK during 1960 election. The consensus is that Nixon was better on radio than on TV (especially during the first debate.). ELG*

22. *The 25th Amendment to the Constitution was adopted in 1967 and provided a remedy to the problem of how to fill a vacancy in either the presidency or the vice presidency. Let's review the history of its use. ELG*

In 1973, VP Spiro Agnew was investigated for receiving kickbacks. This did not involve Watergate. Agnew had four choices; fight any indictment on constitutional grounds, defend himself and go to trial, face impeachment, or resign. Each of these scenarios created a constitutional crisis.

But the 25th Amendment eased the path toward resignation. Instead of perpetuating a crisis, the 25th Amendment offered a remedy. A deal was made, Agnew resigned the vice presidency and pled nolo contendre to one count of tax evasion. There was no trial, no impeachment, no investigation, no involvement by the U.S. Supreme Court

Following Agnew's resignation, Section 2 of the 25th Amendment was activated. *"Whenever there is a vacancy in the office of the Vice President, the President shall nominate a Vice President who shall take office upon confirmation by a majority vote of both Houses of Congress."*

President Richard Nixon nominated Gerald Ford to fill the vacant position. He was soon confirmed by Congress and took office immediately, after taking oath of office. Pretty clear and concise, and easy to put in motion.

In August 1974, there was another serious constitutional crisis. The House Judiciary Committee approved articles of impeachment against President Nixon for his involvement in Watergate. Rather than face certain impeachment Richard Nixon resigned from the presidency onAugust 9, 1974.

Section 1 of the 25th Amendment was activated, and VP Gerald Ford automatically became president. *"In case of the removal of the President from office or of his death or resignation, the Vice President shall become President."* Also, clear and concise. The 25th Amendment was a great remedy for the faults of the original document. But there was then a vacancy in the vice presidency since Ford had vacated that office to become president.

Eleven days later, Section 2 of the 25th Amendment was again activated. *"Whenever there is a vacancy in the office of the Vice President, the President shall nominate a Vice President who shall take office upon confirmation by a majority vote of both Houses of Congress."* President Ford nominated Nelson Rockefeller to be VP, and he was later confirmed by Congress. Upon that confirmation he became VP.

Sections 1 and 2 of the amendment are well written and very clear, and appear to have worked very well. The word devolve did not make an appearance. ELG

23. Seelye, Katherine Q. "Harold N. Bornstein, Trump's Former Personal Physician, dies at 73", *New York Times*, January 14, 2021, pp 53-54. Dr Bornstein stated that President Trump would be the "healthiest president ever."

24. The *Health of the Presidents* by John Bumgarner was the source for most of the information in this chapter.

Chapter 8. Garfield

1. Millard, Candace, *"The Destiny of the Republic"* Doubleday, New York City, 2012

On the morning of his assassination. Garfield did a handstand, playing with his children, ELG

2. Millard, Ibid. Garfield twists after first shot.

3. Millard, Ibid. Dr. Townsend inserts finger.

4. Getien, Larry, "The Inept Doctor who Killed President Garfield," *New York Post* September 22, 2016.

5. Millard, Ibid. Dr. Bliss early days.

6. Ibid.Bliss's probe gets stuck.

7. Ibid. Purvis confronts Bliss.

8. Payne LM., *British Medical Journal*, 1967;4(5570):47-48.

"Guérir quelquefois, soulager souvent, consoler toujours."

This is an old medical maxim, incorrectly attributed to Ambrose Pare. Translation: "to cure sometimes, to relieve often, to comfort always." This has become the dramatic statement of humanism. Take care of the patient. Notice that the word MRI does not make an appearance. ELG

9. Clark, James C. *"The Murder of James A. Garfield"* Jefferson, N.C. McFarland Publishing, January 1, 1993.

10. Millard, Ibid. Conditions in the White House.

11. Ibid. Triumph of Lister in Europe.

12. Ibid. American surgeons.

13. Schwartz, Feather Foster, "The three major inventions of Garfield's Assassination." *Presidential History Blog*, September 16, 2014. https://featherfoster.wordpress.com/2014/09/16/the-three-major-inventions-of-garfields-assassination/

14. Millard, Ibid. Bell invents metal detector.
15. Millard, Ibid. Failure of Bell's experiment.
16. Ibid. Garfield diet.
17. Ibid. Rectal feeding begins.
18. Ibid. Tortured for the Republic.
19. Ibid. Autopsy.
20. Banks, John, "Civil War Veteran's Shocking Souvenir, Bullets in Their Bodies." *HistoryNet*. Accessed 7/4/2022. https://www.historynet.com/civil-war-veterans-shocking-souvenirs-bullets-in-their-bodies/

Chapter 9. Two Paintings

1. "Samuel David Gross" *The Yale Journal of Biology and Medicine*, May 1, 2003 p.128

Dr Gross was quoted as saying, "Little if any faith is placed by any enlightened or experienced surgeon on this side of the Atlantic in the so-called carbolic acid treatment of Professor Lister."

2. Millard, Ibid. p 146.

3. Adams, J. Howe, *History of the Life of D. Hayes Agnew, MD, LLD*, FA Davis Co, Philadelphia and London.

Portrait of Dr Gross (The Gross Clinic), Thomas Eakins 1844-1916, Philadelphia Museum of Art. The Agnew Clinic, Thomas Eakins, University of Pennsylvania Medical School, Philadelphia, 1889.

4. The Agnew Clinic by Thomas Eakins, Annotated by Helle Mathiasen. NYU/Langone Health, Literature, Arts and Medicine Database is a collection of literature, fine art, visual art and performing art annotations created as a dynamic, comprehensive resource for scholars, educators, students, patients, and others interested in medical humanities. It was created by faculty of the New York University School of Medicine in 1993.

Chapter 10: Less than Best Care

1. Markel, Howard. MD "The Excruciating Final Hours of President George Washington." *PBS News,* Dec 14, 2014.

2. Thompson, Mary V., "Death Defied,"*George Washington's Mount Vernon*, Mt. Vernon Ladies' Association. https://www.mountvernon.org/george-washington/death/death-defied-dr-thorntons-radical-idea-of-bringing-george-washington-back-to-life/

3. Wallenborn, White McKenzie, MD. "George Washington's Terminal Illness: A Modern Medical Analysis of the Last Illness and Death of George Washington." *Washington Papers, November 5, 1997.*

4. Dick, Dr. Elisha, "Facts and Observations Relative to the Disease Of Cyanche Trachealis Or Croup," (letter to the editor) *Philadelphia Medical and Physical Journal*, 1809.

5. Hunt, Inez Whitaker, "Nikola Tesla:Serbian-American Inventor." *Encyclopedia Britannica*, January 3, 2022. https://www.britannica.com/biography/Nikola-Tesla.

6. Leary, Thomas; Sholes, Elizabeth, "Buffalo's Pan American Exposition", *Everybody's Magazine,* October 1901 Arcadia Press, 1998

7. Markel, Howard MD, "Would McKinley Have Survived an Assassin's Bullet If He Had a Different Doctor?" *PBS Newshour, September 14, 2019.* https://www.pbs.org/newshour/health/would-mckinley-have-survived-an-assassins-bullet-if-he-had-a-different-doctor

8. Faber, Harold, "The Day of TR's Wild Ride, Sept 4, 1901,"*The NewYork Times,* September 14, 1981,Section B Page 2.

9. "One Day in September"*Roswell Park.org*, April 20, 2016. https://www.roswellpark.org/cancertalk/201604/one-day-september. "When Park walked into the operating room, he noticed that neither Mann nor any of the other surgeons wore surgical gloves, caps, or gowns, nor had they taken steps to disinfect the surgical area. Perspiration from one of the attending surgeons dropped into the president's open wound. The wound was closed without a drain in place."

This observation of Dr. Park confirms the idea that McKinley received less than best care. ELG

Chapter 11: Coverup

1. Millard, Candace, "Change in Chet Arthur." *Destiny of the Nation*, pp300-320

2. Bumgarner, "President Arthur has Glomerulonephritis." *The Health of the Presidents"* p. 132-4.

Arthur's administration had been a very vulnerable time for the presidency and the nation because of his illness and the fact that there was no VP to succeed him. Had Arthur died in office, he would have been succeeded as president by the pro- tempore (PPT).

However, for the first few weeks of Arthur's presidency, the senate PPT office was also vacant! And for the first three months of Arthur's presidency, the position of speaker of the house was also vacant. Just imagine the chaos if Arthur had died during the first three weeks of his presidency.

That situation contributed to changing the 1886 Succession Act. The 1886 Act removed the Speaker and the president pro-tem from the line of succession. Arthur's illness and the vulnerability of the succession process might have also played a role in making the change. Until 1913, US senators were appointed by the state legislatures, so that Arthur's successor in 1881-1885, the senate president would have been a non-elected official. This was contrary to the spirit of a nationally-elected presidency.

The Succession Act of 1947 would change things again and restored the speaker and the. Senate president to the line of succession.. It is important to note that no one has ever become president as a result of the Succession Acts of 1792, 1886, or 1947. ELG

3. Annas, George J.D., "The Public's Right to Know, Health of the President and Presidential Candidates" *New England Journal of Medicine*, October 5, 1995; 333:945-949.

4. Algeo, Matthew, "Presidential Physicians Don't Always Tell the Public the Full Story." *The Atlantic*, October 3, 2020.

Doctors are beholden only to their patients, not to the American people nor to other politicians ELG

5. Algeo, Matthew. "Grover Cleveland's Deadly Secret," *Boat US Magazine,* October 2011.

6. Algeo, Matthew, *The Mag.* March 18, 2017.

7. Renehan A, Lowry JC. "The Oral Tumor's of Two American Presidents: What If They Were Alive Today?"*Journal of the Royal Society of Medicine* 1995 Jul;88(7):377-383.

8. Carlson ER, Reddi SP. "Oral Cancer and United States Presidents." *"Journal of Oral Maxillofacial Surgery."* 2002 Feb; 60(2):1903.

9, Moses JB, Cross W. "When the President Vanished." *Journal of California Dental Association* 1999 April 27(4):325–31.

10. Hoang, HM, O'Leary JP. "President Grover Cleveland's Secret Operation." *The American Surgeon.* 1997 Aug;63(8):758-9.

11. Keen, W.W, "The Surgical Operations on President Cleveland in 1893," *Saturday Evening Post*, September 22, 1917.

Cleveland's cover-up wasn't without casualties. E.J. Edwards, a journalist on the *Philadelphia Press*, wrote about the surgery in August 1893. He had heard rumors of the secret surgery and he located Dr. Hasbrouck, the dentist who administered the anesthesia to Cleveland, and who verified the truthful details of the surgery. The *Philadelphia Press* story was remarkably accurate. It still stands as one of the great scoops in the history of American journalism. But it wasn't perceived that way by the public.

The Cleveland administration categorically denied the charges and launched a smear campaign to discredit and embarrass the reporter, making a public display to destroy his reputation. Newspapers denounced Edwards as a "disgrace to journalism" and a "calamity liar." The tactics were effective. The public sided with Cleveland, who'd built his reputation as the "Honest President." Meanwhile, Edwards' career was essentially ruined.

Cleveland survived the surgery and lived another 15 years,

dying of unrelated GI disease. The cover-up remained in place until 1917, nine years after Cleveland's death. One of the doctors who performed the surgery, W.W. Keen, always regretted how Edwards had been so unjustly maligned.

In 1917, a quarter-century after the operation and a decade after Cleveland's death, Keen finally decided to do something about it. He published a confessional in the *Saturday Evening Post* hoping to "vindicate Mr. Edwards' as a truthful correspondent." Edwards was inundated with congratulatory letters and telegrams, and the outpouring deeply moved him. Edwards even wrote to Keen to thank him for restoring his reputation.

In 1921, Dr. Keen will have a brief second act upon the stage of presidential health when he was one of the doctors who examined the paralyzed FDR at Campobello. He missed the diagnosis of paralytic polio. ELG

Chapter 12. Benefits of Hospitalization

1. Nuland, Sherwin B. "The Doctors' Plague: Germs, Childbed Fever and the Strange Story of Ignac Semmelweis," Norton/Atlas Books, 2003, pp 40–41.

2. Markel, Howard, "Deadly Obstetrical Wards. The Doctor Who Made His Students Wash-Up" *PBSNews,* October 7, 2003 https://www.nytimes.com/2003/10/07/health/the-doctor-who-made-his-students-wash-up.html

3. Neuhauser, D, "Florence Nightingale Gets No Respect, As a Statistician, That Is," *Quality & Safety in Health Care,* vol. 12,4 (2003): 317. doi:10.1136/qhc.12.4.317.

4. Zborowsky T. "The Legacy of Florence Nightingale's Environmental Theory: Nursing Research Focusing on the Impact of Healthcare Environments." *HERD.* Summer;7(4):19-34.

5. Reilly RF. "Medical and surgical care during the American Civil War, 1861–1865." *Proceedings Baylor University Medical Center.* 2016;29(2):138-1.

6. National Park Service, Beit-Aharon, Rebecca, volunteer January 2020.

7. Roberts, CS. "H. L. Mencken and the Four Doctors: Osler, Halsted, Welch, and Kelly." *Proceedings (Baylor University Medical Center)* 2010; 23(4):377–388.

8. Barry, John. "Johns Hopkins, the Big Four," *Great Influenza*, Viking Press, New York, p.p. 34–56.

9. Toledo-Pereyra LH. "The Four Doctors." *Journal of Investigational Surgery.* 2007 Jan–Feb; 20(1):5-7.

10. Lathan SR. "Caroline Hampton Halsted: The First to Use Rubber Gloves in the Operating Room." *Proceedings (Baylor University Medical Center)* 2010;23(4):389-392.

11. Kean, Sam. "The Nurse Who Introduced Gloves to the Operating Room." *Science History Institute.* May 20, 2020. https://www.sciencehistory.org/distillations/the-nurse-who-introduced-gloves-to-the-operating-room

12. Barry, Ibid.

13. Fogg R, Kutikov A, Uzzo RG, Canter D. "How Hugh Hampton Young's Treatment of President Woodrow Wilson's Urinary Retention and Urosepsis Affected the Resolution of World War I." *Journal Urology,* 2011 Sep;186(3):1153-6.

14. Bumgarner, Ibid. 191–194.

15. Herrick JB. "Clinical Features of Sudden Obstruction Of The Coronary Arteries." *JAMA,* 1912; LIX(23):2015–2022.

Chapter 13. Pandemics: Wilson and Trump, Lessons not Learned

1. Barry, John., "*PBS, The Great Influenza*, American Experience , January, 2018

2. "Influenza", CDC.gov, Nov 18, 2021 https://www.cdc.gov/flu/symptoms/index.html

3. Little, Becky, "As the 1918 Flu Emerged, Cover-Up and Denial Helped It Spread," *History.com*, May 26 ,2020. https://www.history.com/news/1918-pandemic-spanish-flu-censorship

4. Craddock, W L. "The Achievements of William Crawford Gorgas." *Military Medicine*, vol. 162,5 (1997): 325-7.

5. Wiggins, Sarah Woolfolk, "William Crawford Gorgas." *Encyclopedia of Alabama*, University of Alabama, February 26, 2007. http://encyclopediaofalabama.org/article/h-1048

6. Barry, John, PBS, *The Great Influenza*, Ibid., Era of Enlightenment

7. Wever PC, van Bergen L. "Death from 1918 Pandemic Influenza During the First World War: A Perspective from Personal and Anecdotal Evidence." *Influenza and Other Respiratory Viruses*. 2014;8(5):538-546.

8. Arnold, Catharine, *"1918, Eyewitness Accounts from the Greatest Medical Holocaust in Modern History."* St. Martin's Press, 2018.

9. Aligne, CA. "Overcrowding and Mortality During the Influenza Pandemic of 1918." *American Journal Public Health*. 2016;106(4):642-644.

10. Davis, Kenneth C, "Philadelphia Threw a WWI Parade that Gave Thousands of Onlookers the Flu." *Smithsonian Magazine,* September 21, 2018.

11. "Battling the Bug: Philadelphia Epidemic." *The Army's Response to Epidemics and Pandemics,* U.S. Army Heritage and Education Center October 2014, U.S. Army War College, Carlisle Barracks, Pa. Public Health Reports / 2010 Supplement 3/Volume 125.

12. Gillett, Mary C — Army historical series photo: "The USS Leviathan was to sail for Europe Sept. 30, 1918, with 9,300 Army troops." Army Medical Department, Washington, D.C., Center of Military History, United States Army.

13. Arnold, Catharine. "Pandemic 1918: Ship of Death," *The History Reader*. St Martin's Press, May 20, 2020. https://www.thehistoryreader.com/world-history/ship-of-death-rates-on-the-rise/

14. Persico, Joseph E. "Nov. 11, 1918: Wasted Lives on Armistice Day," *Army Times,* November 9, 2017

15. Wilensky G. "The Importance of Reestablishing a Pandemic Preparedness Office at the White House." *JAMA Health Forum.* 2020;1(7).

16. Charatan, Fred, "President Bush Announces US Plan for Flu Pandemic." *BMJ* 2005;331(7525): President Bush set three goals: detecting outbreaks, stockpiling vaccines, and having emergency plans in place.

17. Lange, John, "Pandemic Preparedness and Response Under a Different President."

The Hill, 08/10/20.

18. Navarro, J Alexander, "People Gave Up on Flu Pandemic Measures a Century Ago When They Tired of Them." *Michigan Medicine,* April 01, 2021.

19. Byerly CR. "The U.S. Military and the Influenza Pandemic of 1918-1919." *Public Health Report.* 2010;125 Supplement 3:82-91.

Chapter 14. Disaster in Paris / Stalemate in US Senate

1. Marmor, M.D., Michael F. "Wilson, Strokes, and Zebras,"

New England Journal Medicine, Boston, 1982; 307:528-535

August 26, 1982

2. Bumgarner, Ibid. p 280

3. Coll, Steve, "Woodrow Wilson Case of the Flu, and How Pandemics Change History."*The New Yorker,* April 16, 2020.

4. Martello, Thomas "Wilson's Disability Preceded 1919 Stroke, Records Show,"*Washington Post,* November 26, 1990.

5. Barry, John, *The Great Influenza,* New York, Viking, 2004, p 383. Herbert Hoover quote.

6. Barry, John *The Great Influenza,* New York, Viking 2004, pp 382-383

7. Menger RP, Storey CM, Guthikonda B, Missios S, Nanda A, Cooper JM. "Woodrow Wilson's Hidden Stroke of 1919: The Impact of Patient-Physician Confidentiality on United States Foreign Policy " *Neurosurg. Focus.* 2015 Jul;39(1).

8. University of Virginia, *US Presidents*, Woodrow Wilson, Thomas R. Marshall

9. "President Wilson appears before the Senate Foreign Relations Committee." *This Day in History.* History.com. November 16, 2009. https://www.history.com/this-day-in-history/president-wilson-appears-before-the-senate-foreign-relations-committee

10. Miller Center, U of Virginia, *US presidents*, "Woodrow Wilson, Edith Wilson", copyright 2022

11. Connor, Joseph "How Woodrow Wilson's Hidden Illness Left America with No President for Over a Year." *American History Magazine.* June 2017.

12. "Edith Wilson." *First Ladies,* History.com, Updated: March15, 2019, Original: Dec 16, 2009. https://www.history.com/topics/first-ladies/edith-wilson

13. "Edith Wilson." Ibid.

Chapter 15. FDR

1. "What is Polio?" Global Immunization, *Centers for Disease Control* Page last reviewed: September 28, 2021. https://www.cdc.gov/polio/what-is-polio/index.htm

2. Smith, Jean, "FDR." Random House, New York, NY, 2007 p 26.

3. Smith, Ibid. p 218.

4. Burns, Ken, Ward, Geoffrey, "The Roosevelts: An Intimate History." Ken Burns, producer, PBS, 2014.

5. Grubin, David, "FDR," *American Experience,* PBS, 1994. Curtis Roosevelt talks about growing up at the White House.

6. Daughton, Suzanne M. "FDR as Family Doctor: Medical Metaphors and the Role of Physician in the Fireside Chats." American Rhetoric in the New Deal Era, 1932-1945:

A *Rhetorical History of the United States,* Volume 7, edited by Thomas W. Benson, Michigan State University Press, 2006, pp. 33–82.

7. Bliss, Eula. "The Illusion of Natural," *The Atlantic* September 30, 2014.

8. Smith, Ibid. p 216 (progress at Warm Springs, March of Dimes)

9. Bumgarner, John, "The Health of the Presidents," Jefferson, North Carolina, McFarland and Co. pp 208-222.

10. Smith, Ibid. pp 600-601.

11. Bruenn, H G. "Clinical Notes on The Illness and Death of President Franklin D. Roosevelt." *Annals of Internal Medicine*, vol. 72,4 (1970): 579-91. Extensive quotes from the Bruenn article.

12. Steinberg, David, MD. "Dr Lahey's Dilemma," Boston.com, May 29, 2011. http://archive.boston.com/lifestyle/articles/2011/05/29/why_lahey_clinic_founder_frank_lahey_concealed_his_report_on_fdr/

What was hidden in Dr. Lahey's vault?

The founder of the Lahey Clinic chose to conceal his report on President Franklin D. Roosevelt's medical board exam of 1944, until it was finally revealed six decades later, on May 29, 2011. Prior to 2011, the rumors of FDR's health were well circulated around the Boston medical community, complete with a book, autopsy reports, photos of a slice of brain surrounding a melanoma, etc. A small cottage industry formed about these rumors. This article made a fiction of all the false FDR health rumors but did not uncover any new and true information. ELG

13. Ramirez-Moreno, J.M.,Milan Nunez M.V. "Franklin Roosevelt, a Silent Enemy and The Course of History." *Neuro Sciences and History*, Badajoz, 2017, vol 4 (55). A review of the evolvement of modern therapy of hypertension as it relates to the life of FDR.

14. Bhatia, B. B. "On the Use of Rauwolfia Serpentina in High Blood Pressure." *Journal Indian Med. Assoc.* 11: 262–265. 1942.

15. Ward, Geoffrey. "Closest Companion: The Unknown

Story of the Intimate Friend," Simon and Schuster, 2009, 1992 page 404.

16. McCullough, David, *Truman*, New York, Simon and Schuster, 1992, pp292-345.

17. Smith, Ibid. p 219. Faustian Deal.

18. McCullough, Ibid. p 404. Succession Act 1947.

19. How did *The Presidential Succession Act of 1947* come to pass? *Note that the following is only one of several versions of the Truman-Morgenthau conflict. ELG*

The Succession Act of 1886 was in effect in 1945 when Harry Truman became president. The line of succession was President Harry Truman, Secretary of State James Byrne, and Secretary of Treasury Henry Morgenthau. Some thought that after the death of FDR, Morgenthau was a Jew too close to power. He would become president if Byrne and Truman were to be killed during their upcoming trip to Potsdam Germany, perhaps by some diehard Nazis; not an unreasonable notion in July 1945. *Harry Truman had a few anti-Semitic moments in his life but he would not play the anti-Jew card as president. ELG.*

In 1948 Truman showed his true colors about Jews, with his critical support for the creation of the state of Israel, against the vigorous opposition of the US State Department.

The long relationship of Harry Truman and his Jewish friend, Eddie Jacobson, army buddy and business partner, paid off for the Jews of Palestine. ELG

Morgenthau had wanted to go to Potsdam and present his plan to dismantle the German industrial world. Truman was opposed to this plan, as were many others. Before going to Potsdam with Byrne, Truman pressured Morgenthau to resign. There would be several benefits for Truman from this resignation. Most significantly, this resignation effectively ended the Morgenthau Plan. Morgenthau's resignation allowed Truman to replace FDR's man, Morgenthau, with one of his own people, Fred Vinson, in the cabinet.

In retrospect there is a whiff of anti-Semitism about this whole episode. ELG

The resignation gave Truman political room to create a new Succession Law, since Truman wanted his good friend, Sam Rayburn, the speaker of the house to precede the cabinet officers in the line of succession. Besides, Truman felt that elected officials should have priority in the succession process.

In 1947, the Succession Law was changed as Truman had wanted: president, vice president, speaker of the house, president pro tempore of the senate. secretary of state, secretary of the treasury, secretary of war, and other cabinet secretaries, in the order of the founding of their departments.

However, the following phrase is also part of that law "if a cabinet officer is serving due to lack of qualification, disability, or vacancy in the office of speaker or president pro tempore, and, further, if a properly qualified speaker or president pro tempore is elected, then they may assume the acting presidency, supplanting the cabinet officer."

This opens the door for a lot of trouble, namely a serving un-elected president (i.e., a prior secretary of state for example) is unexpectedly challenged by an 88-year-old senator who has just become president pro tem.

To return the senate president to the succession is a monumental blunder, and could cause political chaos. Give Truman a failing grade for this law. This was a gift to his friend Speaker Sam Rayburn. He should have stayed with a bottle of bourbon.

The 1947 Succession law became critical, immediately following Ronald Reagan's shooting in 1981, but more about that later. The 1947 law it is still in place, despite the bungled attempt by Al Haig to change the position of secretary of state in the Succession Act. ELG

20. Lerner, Dr. Barron H. "The Death of Eleanor Roosevelt, Final Diagnosis," *Washington Post*, February 8, 2000.

21. Markel, Howard, "How A Mysterious Ailment Ended Eleanor Roosevelt's Life."<u>Health</u>, *PBS NewsHour,* November 7,

2020. https://www.pbs.org/newshour/health/how-a-mysterious-ailment-ended-eleanor-roosevelts-life

The death of Eleanor Roosevelt is not mentioned at all in our text. But because she was the wife of FDR and perhaps the most famous woman in the world her death from miliary tuberculosis in 1962 may have some relevance for us.

Both of these articles documented the final diagnosis of Eleanor Roosevelt.

This case features some of the factors that are seen in "less than best care" including: medical records were sealed for 25 years; the patient had very good friends on the medical team; and there were too many doctors giving opinions. But that may not be the best conclusion. Mrs. Roosevelt's illness was a very difficult case.

It also illustrates the problems of viewing cases retrospectively. All the possible diagnoses that were considered that took up much of the doctor's time are barely mentioned. In other words, this was a difficult case for doctor and patient and reviewer. Only 25% percent of the time is the diagnosis of miliary tuberculosis made while the patient is still alive.

Mrs. Roosevelt had pleurisy with a lesion in her lung fields in 1919, when she was 35 years old. In light of this past history of chest disease, TB should have been aggressively considered when she first entered hospital with fever cough and abnormal chest X-ray. In 1962, when Mrs. Roosevelt was 78 years old, miliary TB was a treatable disease. It is curious that the Kennedys and the doctors for Eleanor Roosevelt's would have problems considering a diagnosis of TB.

Her doctors narrowed the diagnostic scope too soon (aplastic anemia) and came to the correct diagnosis too late. Mrs. Roosevelt developed aplastic anemia, which may be a diagnosis unto itself, or it may fall under the rubric of pancytopenia, which it did. There may be a six week delay in diagnosis while the TB organism are growing in culture. That delay may be lethal. So, the physicians must be aggressive in initiating diagnosis and anti-TB treatment. Adding prednisone therapy to her treatment increased the risks of TB activating and spreading.

The doctors at Columbia were experts in treating complex cases. But once again I suspect that world famous people do not get the best of care. Sensitive areas such as drug use, sexual history, and alcoholic intake are just a few areas that might not get explored in-depth by attending physicians. Having said all of that, I suspect that was not critical in this case.

She signed out of the hospital against medical advice, and that remains one of the most difficult problems for physicians. The final act of the fickle finger of fate for famous patients was that the TB micro-organisms infecting Mrs, Roosevelt in 1962 were resistant to isoniazid and streptomycin, the standard anti-tuberculous drugs of the time. ELG

Chapter 16. Eisenhower

1. Bumgarner, Ibid. p. 225-6.

2. Bumgarner, Ibid. p. 228

3. Smith, Jean Edward "Eisenhower in War and Peace," Paperback Illustrated, Random House, May 7, 2013, p976.

Smith, Ibid. p10. No combat deaths in eight years.

4. Tolstoy, Leo, *"War and Peace,"* Book IX, Chapter 9, "...the king is the slave of history."

5. Morris, Thomas, "The problem of the punctured Heart," *Revolutions in Surgery,* Wellcome Collection, 2019.

6. Lasby, Clarence G., *Eisenhower's Heart Attack: How Ike Beat Heart Disease and Held on to the Presidency*, First Edition, April 14, 1997 University Press of Kansas; Lawrence, KS.

7. Fortuin, Nicholas."Eisenhower's Heart Attack: How Ike Beat Heart Disease and Held on to The Presidency." Book Review, *New England Journal of Medicine,* June 4, 1998, pp.1703-1704.

"Imagine being the physician called to the bedside of the most powerful and beloved man in the world after he awoke with severe chest pain. This daunting task fell to Dr. Howard M. Snyder when President Dwight Eisenhower summoned him in the early-morning hours of April 24, 1955."

These are the powerful opening sentences of Dr. Dr Fortuin's book review. This humanizes the story and gives a lot of sympathy to Dr. Snyder, who will have the entire world focused upon what he does and how he does it. ELG

8. Herrick JB. "Clinical Features of Sudden Obstruction of the Coronary Arteries,"*JAMA*, 1912; pp :2015–2022:

Roberts, Charles Stewart. "Herrick and Heart Disease." *Clinical Methods: The History Physical and Laboratory Examinations,* edited by H Kenneth Walker et al. 3rd ed.,Butterworths 1990.

9. Eisenhower, Dwight D. "Agreement Between the President and the Vice President as to Procedures in the Event of Presidential Disability." Online by Gerhard Peters and John T. Woolley, *The American Presidency Project* https://www.presidency.ucsb.edu/node/234514

10. Davies, M.K., Hollman, A. "Werner Forssmann." *Heart.* 2000 May, 87 (5):49:

Packy LM, Krischel M, Gross D. "Werner Forssmann: A Nobel Prize Winner and His Political Attitude before and after 1945.*Urology Int.* 2016;96(4):379-85.

Forssman had been a member of the Nazi party since 1932. During World War II Forssman served in the SS as a medical officer, rising to rank of major. He became a prisoner of war, was investigated, not charged, and was released. But he was not allowed to practice medicine for three years. He then resumed practice in a small town in the Black Forest.

In 1956 the unknown Dr. Forssman was given the Nobel Prize in Medicine for his 1929 revolutionary experiment (cardiac catheterization) that opened up the world to the therapeutic innovations of the twenty-first century medicine.

11. Norum, Jan, et al.Calculating the 30 Day Survival Rate in Acute Myocardial Infarction: Should we Use the Treatment Chain or the Hospital Catchment Model? " *Heart International,*vol. 12, February, 2017.

12. Lee, Thomas H. MD. "Seizing the Teachable Moment:

Lessons from Eisenhower's Heart Attack," *New England Journal Medicine*, October 20, 2020. "One reason to study history is to avoid repeating past mistakes; another is to understand what went right."

Chapter 17A. The Legend of John Kennedy

1. Dallek, Robert, "The Medical Ordeals of John Kennedy," *Atlantic*, December 2002. *This was my main source of reliable information about Kennedy's medical history. ELG*

2. Macchia D, Lippi D, Bianucci R, Donell S. "President John F Kennedy's Medical History: Celiac Disease and Autoimmune Polyglandular Syndrome Type 2." *Postgrad Med J*. 2020 Sep; 96(1139): pp543-549.

The genetics of the autoimmune polyglandular syndrome, Type II have only recently been revealed. It is a rare recessive familial disorder. Supporting evidence for this diagnosis are twofold: JFK's sister had adrenal insufficiency, his son had thyroid disease. To support the diagnosis, we need to assume that JFK's bowel disease was celiac disease, which is associated with APS-2

3. Glyn, JH "The Discovery of Cortisone: A Personal Memory." *BMJ*, 1998; 317(7161): 822A.

4. Plotkin, Stephen. "Sixty Years Later, the Story of PT-109 Still Captivates" *Prologue Magazine*, Summer 2003, Vol. 35, No. 2. Plotkin was an archivist at the JFK library, but *Prologue* is the journal of the US National Archives. *The story of PT 109 is truly remarkable. ELG*

5. Nomura K, Demura H, Saruta T. "Addison's Disease in Japan: Characteristics and Changes Revealed in a Nationwide Survey." *Intern Med*. 1994 Oct; 33(10):602-6.

6. Part TG, Dowdy JT. "John F. Kennedy's Back: Chronic Pain, Failed Surgeries, and the Story of Its Effects on His Life and Death." *J Neurosurg Spine*. 2017 Sep; 27(3): 247–255. *This is interesting and unique article told from the perspective of neurosurgeons and others who do spinal surgery. They focused on the indi-*

cations or lack of them for JFK's early surgeries. They never commented upon the presence of unilateral sacroileitis in a young man, and how that could become a link to additional medical history. Rheumatologists have long noted that unilateral sacroileitis might be a harbinger of more generalized disease, such as inflammatory bowel disease, psoriasis, ankylosing spondylitis etc. ELG

7. Nichols, James A. "The Management of Adrenal Cortical Insufficiency During Surgery," *Archives of Surgery, 1955,*

pp 732,742

8. Bumgarner, Ibid. Response to Bobby Kennedy's lies about Addison's disease.

9. Fisher, Eddie. *Been There, Done That: An Autobiography*, St. Martin's Press, New York, NY, 1999.

10. Carlson, Peter. "How 'Doctor Feelgood' Almost Drove John F. Kennedy to the Brink of Nuclear Disaster," *History Net,* June 29, 2011. https://www.historynet.com/jack-kennedy-dr-feel good/.

Dr Jacobson injected JFK with amphetamines during house calls at the White House, Hyannis Port, and Palm Beach. ELG

11. Bumgarner p254. Dr Raymond Adams is quoted

Chapter 17B. JFK Assassination

There are hundreds if not thousands of articles about the assassination of JFK. I found a few that focused mainly upon the medical care and not on conspiracies. The 1992 JAMA articles purportedly supported the Warren Commission, but please come to your own conclusions.

The National Archives contains both the Warren Commission Report and the House Assassination Committee report. These reports reach different conclusions about the number of shooters, the number of bullets and have different conclusions about shooters and conspiracy.

It is difficult not to be attracted to these brightly colored conspiracy threads, true or false. The wary weaver tries hard to reject them and to stay with the basic strands of medical history.

Therefore, there is very little about conspiracies, and most of the narrative is about JFK and his medical history and medical care. ELG.

1. *Most of the information in chapter 17B can be found in a few sources. ELG*

These include the following:
National Archives, JFK Assassination Records
Three articles from JAMA 1992.
Two articles from New York Times
Two references pertaining to the details of the flight back from Dallas
National Archives, JFK Assassination Records
Warren Commission report
House Assassination Committee report
Report from National Archives conspiracies.

Appendix 9: Autopsy Report and Supplemental Report. The autopsy Report has now been digitized. This appendix (pages 538 through 546) reproduces commission exhibit No. 387.

The three articles from JAMA 1992 are accounts by the treating physicians and the pathologists, and are the second major source of medical information:

1. Breo, Dennis. "Dallas Docs Recall their Memories" *JAMA*, vol 267, pp 2804-2807.

2. Breo, Dennis. "JFK's Death-The Plain Truth from the MDs Who Did the Autopsy"*JAMA*, 1992; 267

3. Lundberg, George. Editorial, *JAMA,* 1992, vol.268 pp1736-8.

The pathologists were persuaded to talk about the JFK autopsy by editor of JAMA, Dr. George D. Lundberg. This was part of his seven-year effort to answer lingering questions about the Kennedy autopsy and to help rebut conspiracy theories.

Reporting in *JAMA*, two pathologists at the autopsy of John F. Kennedy broke a long silence and reported that the Kennedy's adrenal glands were found but were represented only by tiny fragments of adrenal tissue. This establishes, that

Kennedy did suffer for many years from adrenal insufficiency or Addison's disease; contrary to the repeated denials and cleverly worded cover stories issued from Kennedy, his family, and his aides,

A third pathologist, Dr. Pierre Finck, now says that the Kennedy family at first did not want the pathologists to examine Kennedy's abdominal cavity. The adrenals, usually two in number, are located within the abdomen, sitting on top of each kidney.

This report showed without a doubt that JFK had Addison's disease, and the Kennedys took their cover-up attempts into the morgue. This was highlighted by attempts of the Kennedys to prevent an autopsy that would include the abdominal cavity where the adrenals are located. This cover-up by the Kennedys defies logic. ELG

2. Walker, Noel, "Demolition of Parkland" NBC Broadcast July 22, 2022

3. Breo, Dennis."Dallas Docs Recall Their Memory" *JAMA*, vol 267, 1992. pp 2804-2807.

4. Breo, Ibid.

5. Breo, Ibid.

6. Breo, Ibid.

7. Breo, Ibid.

8. Martin, Douglas. "Obituary of Dr Earl Rose," *New York Times,* May 2, 2012.

This is a standalone article from the point of view of a well-placed observer/participant.

Then there are two references that detail of the flight to Washington DC, ELG

9. Jones, Chris. "The flight from Dallas" *Esquire,* October 1, 2013.

10. Graff, Garret. "Angel Is Airborne" *Washingtonian,*October 15, 2013.

11. Graff, Ibid.

Returning to the JAMA articles

12. Breo, Dennis, "JFK's Death, The Plain Truth from The MDs Who Did the Autopsy,"

JAMA, 1992., vol 267.

13. Breo, Ibid.

14. Breo, Ibid.

15. Breo. Ibid.

Second of two articles from New York Times

16. Altman, Lawrence K. "Disturbing News of Kennedy's Secret Illness," *New York Times*, October 6, 1992. This block buster is also about the missing adrenal glands.

17. Graff, Ibid.

18. What has become of Trauma Room 1? It has been demolished. Six years ago, the National Archives moved any remaining artifacts from its Fort Worth facility and sent the Parkland crates to underground storage in Lenexa, Kansas.

Chapter 18. Shooting Reagan.

1. Siang Yong Tan, Merritt, Christopher." Charles Richard Drew (1904–1950): Father of blood banking," *Singapore Med Journal.* 2017, Oct; 58(10): 593–594.

Unfortunately, Drew's death became an example of the Liberty Valence syndrome. "When the legend becomes the fact, print the legend" ELG

Drew was severely injured in an auto accident in 1950, at night on the back roads of North Carolina. All agree that he was taken to a local hospital. And now the fiction/memory writers take over:

He was denied admission to a white only hospital or

He was admitted but not treated or

He was treated but not given any blood or plasma or

He died because of poor care

This makes great story telling. The black man who invented blood banking died because he was denied blood transfusion. This legend was repeated many times by prominent black dignitaries. But the legend is contrary to the facts. ELG

The facts are more mundane but just as deadly. Dr. Drew was in a severe auto accident and was initially trapped inside the auto. He was taken to a local hospital in Alamance County which was segregated, but did treat Afro-Americans. There was a black clinician on Drew's treatment team. He was immediately given plasma but died within 30 minutes of entry into the hospital.

The legend of the accident does give voice to the unspoken true history of ordinary black Americans who were denied medical care in the days of Jim Crow. The story of denial of care has so much powerful irony, that it has endured as the story that black Americans remember.

"When the legend becomes the fact, print the legend" In this instance, the legend has illuminated the true story of the denial of medical care for thousands of Afro-Americans during Jim Crow. ELG

2. Alivizatos, Peter A. "Dwight Emary Harken, MD, An All-American Surgical Giant: Pioneer Cardiac Surgeon, Teacher Mentor." *Proceedings (Baylor University Medical Center) vol 31, 4, 554-557*

3. *Cleveland Plain Dealer,* April 13, 1981.

4. Clark, David E, "R A Crowley, the Golden Hour, the Momentary Pause, and the Third Space," The American Surgeon, vol 83,12 (2017):1401-1406.

5. "Remembering Assassination Attempt on Ronald Reagan,"
Larry King Live, CNN, Aired March 30, 2001

6. Allen, Richard V. "The Day Reagan Was Shot," *Atlantic Monthly,* April 2001.

The author reveals previously undisclosed transcripts of the deliberations in the White House Situation Room while Reagan was undergoing emergency surgery.

The first FBI act of incompetence was informing the surgeons of the incorrect bullet caliber. It was a .22 caliber bullet and not a .38. Their next sign of incompetence was to announce that Jim Brady was dead, when he was still alive. He had a partial recovery and lived until 2014.

Their final act was their performance in Nashville, when they first encountered John Hinckley. That completed their trifecta of incompetence. The would-be assassin Hinckley had followed President Carter on the campaign trail, looking for an opportunity to kill him. That was not to be in Nashville, so Hinckley bought airline tickets for New York City where Carter was to appear the next day.

At the airport, Hinckley was stopped. Three loaded guns were found in his baggage, his tickets for New York were also found, and he was detained by the local police. The FBI, who had jurisdiction in cases involving interstate travel, was then notified. In an incredible display of incompetence, the FBI told the police to release Hinckley, and did not put him under surveillance.

A young man seems to be following President Carter on the campaign trail. He is found to have three loaded weapons with him. Shouldn't this be worrisome and a potential threat to Carter? Aren't you concerned? ELG

7. National Archives. Gov

8. Shirley, Craig, Heubusch, John, Larry King Special January 10, 1991. Ten years later on CNN, President Reagan didn't appear to have Alzheimer's while on the TV show

9. Altman, Lawrence MD. "Reagan and Alzheimer's" Following Path His Mother Travelled, She Also had Alzheimer's," *New York Times*, November 8, 1994.

GLOSSARY

- ***abscess***, *collection of infected material in tissues, organs, or circumscribed spaces*
- ***Aedes Aegyptii***, *species of mosquito associated with Yellow Fever*
- ***amphetamines***, *central nervous system stimulant*
- ***amyloidosis***, *group of diseases with abnormal protein deposition. causing disruption of function.*
- ***anasarca***, *generalized swelling of the body*
- ***anhedonia***, *taking little or no pleasure from life's activities.*
- ***anticoagulant***, *substance that inhibits clotting of the blood*
- ***antiseptic,*** *substance that destroy harmful microorganisms or inhibit their activity*
- ***anti-toxin,*** *serum from immunized animals used against specific bacterial toxins.*
- ***apocryphal,*** *well known but not true*
- ***ascites***, *accumulation or retention of free fluid within the peritoneal cavity*

- **asepsis,** *prevention of access by infecting organisms to area of potential infection.*
- **atrial fibrillation,** *disorder of cardiac rhythm with rapid, irregular atrial impulses*
- **auscultation,** *listening for sounds within the body, usually the heart*
- **axillary,** *area of body where the arm meets the chest and forms a cavity(arm pit)*
- **bronchiectasis,** *persistent abnormal dilatation of the bronchial tubes*
- **calomel,** *white tasteless compound usually containing mercury used as purgative*
- **camphor,** *a liniment, a mild analgesic*
- **carbolic acid,** *antiseptic and disinfectant active against a range of micro-organisms*
- **cathartic,** *agents that promote/ease defecation by accelerating passage of feces*
- **cartography,** *the process or skill of making maps*
- **cerebral hemorrhage,** *bleeding within the substance of the brain*
- **cholecystectomy,** *surgical removal of the gall bladder*
- **cholera,** *acute diarrheal disease can lead to severe dehydration, rice water stools*
- **colic,** *paroxysms of pain, usually the abdominal region may occur elsewhere*
- **colitis,** *inflammation of the colon, the large intestine*
- **compos mentos,** *of sound mind*
- **CPR,** *Cardio Pulmonary Resuscitation*
- **Crohn's disease,** *chronic inflammatory disease of intestine usually involving terminal ileum*
- **croup,** *condition characterized by barking cough, hoarseness and stridor*
- **delirium,** *an acute mental disorder with confused thinking and disrupted attention*

- *digitalis,* powerful cardio-tonic that increases the force of myocardial contraction;
- *diphtheria,* bacterial infection of upper airways, may cause death by obstructed air way caused by pseudomembrane. Associated with carditis and neuritis
- *edema*, excess accumulation of fluid
- *electro-cautery,* application of an electric current, in order to destroy tissue.
- *encephalopathy,* brain damage of dysfunction
- *enteric*, of, relating to, or affecting the intestines
- *entomology,* branch of zoology that deals with insects
- *fistula,* abnormal connection between two internal organs, or between an internal organ and the surface of the body
- *glomerulonephritis*, inflammation of small blood vessels of glomeruli, the filtering system of the kidneys
- *Guillain Barre*, acute inflammatory autoimmune neuritis causing by demyelination in peripheral nerves and nerve roots; often preceded by a viral infection,
- *hemoptysis*, bronchial hemorrhage manifested with spitting of blood
- *hemorrhagic,* to bleed in a very fast and uncontrolled way
- *heparin,* powerful anti-coagulant, found in leeches
- *herd immunity,* protection offered by the combined immune status of the group
- *homeopathic,* system for treating illnesses, using minimal amounts of substances, that in larger amounts produce symptoms of the illnesses in healthy people
- *homeostasis,* stable state of equilibrium, of harmony among interdependent concepts
- *hydrotherapy,* use of water in the treatment of disease or injury
- *hyperthyroidism,* excessive activity of the thyroid gland, with increased metabolic rate,

- **hypothermia,** *subnormal temperature of the body*
- **immunity,** *condition of being able to resist a particular disease or toxin*
- **immunotherapy,** *treatment or prevention of disease by increasing immune system function by administration of vaccines or antibodies*
- **inferior vena cava,** *great vein that drains lower half of body, enters right atrium of the heart*
- **internal milieu,** *product of the organism and controlled by it, permits the organism to maintain desirable conditions for cells to function, despite external factors operating to disrupt or destroy homeostatic balance.*
- **jaundice,** *yellow discoloration of skin due elevated blood levels of bilirubin; classic sign of liver disease*
- **malaria ,** *disease cause when the bite of the anopheles mosquito inject the malaria parasite into its victims.*
- **Marfan's syndrome,** *genetic disorder affecting the skeleton, the eyes and the heart. People are very tall and thin, see paintings El Greco, Modigliani*
- **melanoma,** *malignancy derived from cells capable of forming the pigment, melanin,*
- **metastatic,** *having spread from primary site of disease to another part of the body*
- **microbe,** *organisms that are too small to be seen without only a microscope*
- **micro- organism,** *living organism only seen under a microscope*
- **murmur,** *abnormal heart sounds heard during auscultation*
- **neck dissection,** *major surgery done to remove lymph nodes that contain cancer*
- **nephrotoxic,** *poisonous to the kidney*
- **neuropathy,** *damage, disease or dysfunction of one or more peripheral nerves,*

Glossary

- ***nitrous oxide**, colorless, odorless gas that is used as an anesthetic and analgesic.*
- ***opiates**, any natural or synthetic derivative of opium or morphine*
- ***osteomyelitis**, Infection of the bone, usually bacterial, occasionally tuberculous*
- ***ovarian**, pertaining to the ovary, organs that produce eggs and female hormones*
- ***paleontology**, the study of the forms of life existing in pre historic times*
- ***panacea**, a remedy for all ills or difficulties: cure-all*
- ***pancreatic necrosis**, a process leading to cell death of the pancreas gland*
- ***paracentesis**, procedure in which fluid is withdrawn from a body cavity via a cannula, needle, or other hollow instrument*
- ***paranoia**, chronic mental disorders with a development of an unshakeable and permanent delusional system, with preservation of clear, orderly thinking.*
- ***pericarditis**, inflammation of the serous sac surrounding the heart and great vessels.*
- ***peritoneum**, the parietal peritoneum covers the inside of the abdominal wall and the visceral peritoneum covers the bowel, the mesentery, and some organs.*
- ***petit mal epilepsy**, a seizure disorder with sudden cessation of ongoing activity usually no loss of postural tone. Rhythmic blinking of eyelids, lasts 5-10 seconds.*
- ***phlebitis**, inflammation of veins*
- ***phlegm**, calmness in a difficult or unpleasant situation, one of the four humors, considered to be cold and moist, apathetic coldness or intrepid coolness*
- ***polymath**, person of encyclopedia learning/knowledge*
- ***polyp**, protrusions from any mucous membrane.*
- ***Polypharmacy**, simultaneous use of multiple drugs in one person*

- ***post mortem**, something occurring after death*
- ***pox**, viral disease characterized by pustules or eruptions, also a curse*
- ***puerperal**, diseases within six-to-eight-weeks following labor and delivery.*
- ***purgative**, substances that causes the bowels to empty*
- ***pulmonary embolism**, blood clot from periphery that has traveled to the lung*
- ***quarantine**, kept away from others to prevent a disease from spreading(40 days)*
- ***quinine**, an antimalarial drug since 1633, and derived from bark of cinchona tree*
- ***rabies**, acute viral infectious disease of central nervous system spread by virus-laden saliva of bites inflicted by rabid animals.*
- ***rales**, abnormal sounds heard upon auscultation over respiratory tract areas.*
- ***resuscitate** to revive from apparent death or from unconsciousness; also revitalize*
- ***retinal hemorrhage**, bleeding from the vessels of the retina*
- ***rhonchi**, whistling or snoring sound heard on auscultation, when the airways are partly obstructed*
- ***Rickettsia**, bacteria that are intracellular parasites of arthropods (as lice or ticks) and when transmitted to humans cause various diseases (as typhus)*
- ***Salmonella**, bacteria toxic for humans, causing fevers, gastroenteritis, and food poisoning, the most common clinical manifestation*
- ***schizophrenia**, severe mental illness characteristically marked by a retreat from reality with delusions, hallucinations, and emotional disharmony*
- ***sepsis**, systemic reaction (fever, hypoxemia, low urine flow) resulting from the spread of bacteria or their toxins from a focus of infection;*

- *sequelae,* an aftereffect of a disease, condition, or injury, a secondary result
- *sickling,* an abnormal red blood cell of crescent shape, resistant to malaria
- *string sign,* localized narrowing of the small intestine, diagnostic of Crohn's'
- *subdural Hematoma,* blood clot located between the skull and the surface of the brain
- *sphygmomanometer,* device that measures blood pressure
- *syphilis,* chronic contagious usually sexually transmitted (sometimes congenital) disease caused by a spirochete. If left untreated produces rashes, and systemic lesions in a three stage clinical course over many years —primary syphilis (genitalia), secondary syphilis (skin), tertiary syphilis (heart, brain)
- *Stelazine,* an anti-psychotic medication
- *streptococcal,* common bacterial infection: sore throat, rheumatic fever, nephritis.
- *tracheotomy,* emergency operation in which an incision is made in the trachea (windpipe) allowing a person to breathe.
- *triage,* the sorting out and classification of patients or casualties to determine priority of need and proper place of treatment.
- *thoracic,* pertaining to the thorax, the chest
- *thrombolytic,* ability to destroy or dissolve thrombi in blood vessels or bypass grafts.
- *thrombophlebitis,* inflammation of a vein associated with thrombus formation.
- *thrombosis,* formation and development of a thrombus.
- *thrombus,* clot of blood formed within a blood vessel and remaining attached
- *Tuinal,* an effective medicine for insomnia, but highly addictive.

- ***typhoid,*** *an acute systemic febrile infection caused by Salmonella typhi*
- ***vasoconstriction,*** *episodic narrowing of the blood vessels without anatomic change*
- ***venous,*** *relating to the veins*
- ***ventricular aneurysm,*** *abnormal blood-filled bulge of the heart wall resulting from weakening or disease of the heart wall*
- ***Vibrio,*** *type of microorganism that causes cholera*
- ***Virginia snakeroot,*** *a poisonous plant; when dairy cows feed on this, their milk become toxic. This causes a disease in humans called milk illness, and was the cause of death of Abraham Lincoln's mother, Nancy Hanks Lincoln.*
- ***virulent,*** *malignant, poisonous, very infectious*
- ***Zika,*** *viral illness cause by mosquito bite, fetal toxicity*

LIST OF IMAGES AND ATTRIBUTIONS

1. **Way West: Historical Wilderness Road Map** Philadelphia and Baltimore to Cumberland, GapMatt Holly July 1, 2016; US National Park Service, public domain
2. **First Major Expansion from Appalachians to the Mississippi;** The 1783 Treaty of Paris recognized the Mississippi River as the new western boundary of the US. The US in 1790, National Atlas of the US, 1970 edition.
3. **Life cycle Aedes mosquito;** Centers for Disease Control (CDC,) March 5 2020, public domain
4. **Lewis and Clark Expedition;** Author: Victor van Werhooven, May 22, 2014; public domain
5. **Antiseptic Surgery Using Carbolic Acid Spray;** Lister in center holding scissors "Antiseptic surgery its principles, practices and results,"1882, William Watson Cheynne.

6. **LBJ receiving bad news from Vietnam**; President Lyndon B. Johnson listens to tape sent by Captain Charles Robb from Vietnam, 07/31/1968", Jack E. Kightlinger, Photographer (National Archives Identifier: 192617); Collection LBJ-WHPO: White House Photo Office Collection, 11/22/1963 - 01/20/1969; Lyndon Baines Johnson Library; National Archives and Records Administration
7. **Shooting James Garfield;** Images of American Public History web site, public domain; A. Burghaus and C. Upham, engravers; 1881, published in *Frank Leslie's Illustrated Newspaper*
8. **Garfield's autopsy**; Autopsy report, From Official Bulletins and Autopsy 1881
9. *The Gross Clinic*, **by Thomas Eakins, 1875,** The Philadelphia Museum of Art;
10. *The Agnew Clinic*, **by Thomas Eakins, 1889,** University of Pennsylvania medical school, Philadelphia, public domain
11. **Pan Am Exposition, Buffalo, New York, 1901;** Panorama View with The Electric Tower; University of Buffalo: http://ublib.buffalo.edu/libraries/exhibits/panam/art/architecture/panorama.html; unidentified photographer, from "The Latest and Best Views of the Pan-American Exposition", Buffalo, N.Y.: Robert Allen Reid, 1901; public domain
12. **An obese Grover Cleveland (seated,) awaits surgery on board the Oneida;** Grover Cleveland on board the private yacht Oneida, site of his secret cancer operation during his term as president, 1893. New Jersey State Park Service, Grover Cleveland Birthplace
13. **FDR swimming in Pool at Warm Springs;** FDR in the pool at Warm Springs with others, circa 1930. FDR Library Photograph Collection, NPx 48-

22:4014(3) https://nara.getarchive.net/media/franklin-delano-roosevelt-swimming-in-a-pool-at-warm-springs-georgia-45ef66?zoom=true

14. **On the road in Georgia**; Roosevelt, Franklin D. (Franklin Delano), 1882-1945; *Franklin D. Roosevelt, Otis Moore, and Ed Doyle in Warm Springs, Georgia*; Franklin D. Roosevelt Library Public Domain Photographs, 1882 - 1962 (National Archives Identifier:1184) Series: Franklin D. Roosevelt Library Public Domain Photographs, compiled 1882 - 1962 (National Archives Identifier: 195301)
15. **The last portrait of President Franklin D. Roosevelt,** taken on April 11, 1945, one day before his death; FDR Library, unknown author; public domain.
16. **Jackie at LBJ's swearing in ceremony**; LBJ sworn in as President Nov 22, 1963 Air Force One, Jackie Kennedy by his side; Photographer Cecil Stoughton, National Archives, LBJ Library) Public domain
17. **The Reagans post-op in hospital**; George Washington Hospital 1981; Reagan Library, public domain
18. Cover image: **Professors Welch, Halsted, Osler and Kelly, aka The Four Doctors, by John Singer Sargent, 1906;** owned by Johns Hopkins University, (Baltimore); resides in the Welch Medical Library. It is in the public domain per Mr Tim Vishnevski, library archivist.

BIBLIOGRAPHY

Adams, Henry, *History of the United States,* New York, Literary Classics of America, 1986

Allen, Richard "The Day Reagan Was Shot", Atlantic Monthly, Boston, 2002

Annas, George. "Health of the President and Presidential Candidates The Public's Right to Know", New England Journal of Medicine, Boston, 1995

Atkinson, Rick. *The British Are Coming,* New York, Henry Holt, 2019

Barry, John. *The Great Influenza,* New York, Viking, 2004

Belofsky, Nathan. *Strange Medicine,* New York, Tarcher Perigree, 2013

Beschloss, David, *The Conquerors, New York,* Simon and Schuster, 2002

Bruenn, Howard. "Clinical Notes on the Illness and Death of President Franklin D. Roosevelt,"

Philadelphia, Annals of Internal Medicine 1970,

Buchanan, John, *The Road to Charleston,* Charlottesville, University of Virginia Press, 2019

Bumgarner, John. *The Health of the American Presidents,* Jefferson N.C. McFarland, 2003

Carmichael, David W. *Reputation in Flames,* Amazon, 2013

Chernow, Ron, *Grant,* New York, Penguin, 2017

Connolly AJ, Finkbeiner WE, Ursell PC, Davis RL. Legal, Social, and Ethical Issues. *Autopsy Pathology: A Manual and Atlas.* 2016;15-23. doi:10.1016/B978-0-323-28780-7.00002-0

Dallek, Robert, "The Medical Ordeals of John Kennedy," Boston, Atlantic Monthly, Dec. 2002

Dean, John W, *Warren Harding,* New York, Times Book, 2004

Encyclopedia Britannica Online, Chicago, 1994

Fenn, Elizabeth. *Pox Americana,* New York, Hill and Wang, 2001

Fischer, David Hacker. *Washington's Crossing,* Press, Oxford, Oxford University, 2004

Fisher, Eddie. *Been There, Done That,* New York, St Martin's Press, 1999

Fitzharris, Lindsey. *The Butchering Art,* New York, Farrar, Straus and Giroux, 2017

Graff, Garrett M. *"Angel is Airborne"* Washington DC, Washingtonian, 2103

Katz, Catherine Grace, *The Daughters of Yalta,* Houghton, Mifflin, Harcourt, Boston 2020

Lasby, Clarence. *Eisenhower's Heart Attack:"How Ike Beat Heart Disease And Held On To The Presidency"* Lawrence Kansas, University Press of Kansas, 1997

MacMillan, Margaret. *Paris 1919*, New York, Random House, 2001
McCullough, David. *1776*, New York, Simon and Schuster, 2005
McCullough, David. *The Path Between the Seas,* New York, Simon and Schuster, 1977
McCullough, David. *Truman*, New York, Simon and Schuster, 1992
Millard, Candace. *Destiny of the Republic.* New York, Doubleday, 2011
Oldstone, Michael. *Viruses Plagues and History,* Oxford U.K., Oxford University Press,1998
Oshinsky, David. *Bellevue*, New York, Penguin, 2016
Phillips, Kevin, *1775.* New York, Penguin 2013
Robenalt, James. *The Harding Affair*, London, Palgrave MacMillan 2009
Smith, Jean, *FDR.* New York, Random House, 2008
Smith, Jean. *Eisenhower in War and Peace,* New York, Random House, 2013
Snowden, Frank. *Epidemics and Society.* New Haven, Yale University Press, 2019
Starr, Paul. *The Social Transformation of American Medicine,* New York, Basic Books, 1982

ACKNOWLEDGMENTS

This book has had a long gestation period. Perhaps it began the first or second time that I read the *Microbe Hunters* by Paul de Kruif. Maybe it began during the second year of medical school when I began to meet patients and record their medical histories.

Many thanks to the thousands of patients, who told me their stories, over the years, as I learned to listen closely. What a rich and rewarding experience that was. My patients were a broad spectrum of the world, my living library, which I cherished. Farmers, lobstermen, homemakers, professors, laborers, anthropologists, gold miners, artists, cops and firefighters. It was so interesting. Probably most physicians who practiced primary care internal medicine feel that way. What a privilege to have provided some medical care for them. Medicine and medical history were so exciting and I loved it.

I would like to give a special thanks to the Veteran's Administration for the opportunity to practice medicine in the VA. It was and is an honor to have been a physician for our veterans.

My worst moment as an intern was the following: Once again at the Syracuse VA, a young man with Hodgkin's disease began to bleed, and within a minute blood was pouring out of his mouth. Very quickly, I was covered from head to toe with his blood. It was in my mouth, my nose, my hair, my eyes, in my shoes, everywhere. My desperate attempts to stop the bleeding were futile. The patient died within minutes, after which I ran outside screaming. There I was incoherent, covered with blood, wrapped around the base of the VA's flagpole. Medical internship was like combat, and I had earned my stripes. The chief of medicine gave me off an extra hour to go home and take a shower and have breakfast, and I returned to work.

I learned to put things into perspective. Nothing that I endured as a medical intern, could compare with the horror of combat.

Dr. Norman Levinsky had taught the lesson, to go all the way for our patients, do everything possible, and leave no stone unturned in seeking the truth. No matter the outcome we were always asking, "Did I do enough? Was I smart enough?"

And when death came to our patients, and colleagues rallied to support me, I joined a long line of physicians going back thousands of years. I need to acknowledge all the support from my comrades in caring. That has helped to sustain me over the years.

On occasion, death would come gently, and I softly cried, holding the eighteen-year-old T.P. in my arms for several hours, as he passed away from metastatic osteogenic sarcoma. Cancer almost always won.

I began to write about patients—imaginary and real. This became an anodyne for all the trauma of medicine. The following is a true story that I first recorded almost fifty years ago. When I was in private practice, a man named Charlie became my patient. He lived alone and was a veteran of World War I. He was beginning to lose weight, and I saw him, trying to find out what was happening. What was happening was a large inoperable gastric cancer. A desperate search for something therapeutic to do came up empty.

On one memorable day he came to my office. He was so emaciated that he had trouble holding up his pants. But he brought me a manila envelope which contained a black and white photograph of his World War I air force squadron. There was Charlie standing tall next to his plane, with his leather flying coat, goggles, leather cap, and long white scarf encircling his neck, completing the image of a gallant knight of the sky. Charlie pointed out to me the two pilots in the squadron who did not survive that September morning in 1918. They were shot down and killed.

I had a hard time with these images. Who was Charlie, the flyboy with his long white scarf, or the old man trying to hold up his pants? That's all that I have left, my competing images of Charlie. The young airmen weren't dead, they were alive forever in the photo, more than their memory, there was their image, like the historical images of the painted Grecian urns. Medicine is a demanding mistress, and the demands were immediate. Stop day dreaming and try to keep Charlie comfortable. When things unravel, they seem to move pretty fast, and Charlie died a few days later. A previously unknown sister, from a thousand miles away, took Charlies remains with her, before I said goodbye.

Words were failing me. I wanted to capture history in my writing, but history seems to have caught me in a morass. But I wanted to keep writing.

For all my medical friends, who have toiled in the fields, thanks for sharing the challenges, the disbelief, the outrage, the wonder of it all. Telling dark humorous stories is a survival technique that helped to cope with all the suffering humanity that we encountered. I wanted to preserve the unique perspective of the front-line doc, and I have endeavored to keep that perspective, my voice, in the narrative.

After retirement, I joined Osher lifelong learning, at Brandeis, (BOLLI) and began to read a lot of American history. I was eventually given the opportunity to make a few presentations at BOLLI, thanks to Bernie and Elaine Reisman, both of whom were Brandeis scholars and wonderful human beings. My presentations became five-week courses; the most successful of them was the Medical History of the Presidents.

My partner Eileen and I spent the winter months in San

Diego, where I attended many lectures on American history at Osher UCSD, presented by Dan Dinan. He was a great public speaker, with so many great stories, mostly about recent American history. I was absorbed by his story telling techniques, like partaking of a master class.

I could mimic his style but never could replicate his fund of knowledge. Nevertheless, I began to lecture. My great thanks to Admiral Steve Clarey, chair curriculum committee at Osher, UCSD. He gave me the opportunity and the encouragement to make my presentations. Several friends said there was a book in the lecture series on the Health of the Presidents.

In my naivety, I began to sort my lecture notes into the form of a book. That did not seem so hard, but what had I produced, was a series of lecture notes. Very irreverent, somewhat risqué. What was I writing?

My college fraternity brother Joel Jayson was a great help. He turned me to pursue a more serious enterprise, and showed me the many failings of my book. A lecture is not a chapter in a book. They have different modes and rhythm of presentation. Thanks Joel for reading hundreds of pages of mediocre literature. I still didn't know how to write well, but I began to appreciate the difference between good and bad. I increased my investment in time and effort. I read many of the great contemporary historians, and noted their skills at storytelling, especially their ease at placing you at the scene of the story.

Enter Stephen Douglas Royer, attorney, vacation neighbor and "anchor of the nation." He bought a lot of encouragement, good ideas and living proof that Republicans and Democrats can co-exist, and have some fun doing that.

I still thought I had the potential for writing a good book, and so I gave a copy to my friend Debra Ettenberg, erstwhile English teacher. She said that the book was interesting, but unfortunately was not well written.

I re-read Strunk and White, my fellow Cornell alumni and strove to improve my grammar. I then began to think how I was going to print this book; self-publish like my friend Dr. Bob Mindelzun, but he was so much smarter than me and I doubted I could duplicate his effort.

Several months ago, I spoke with my friend Rachel Falk. She renewed my confidence, by telling me how things got done, how to get my text to a publisher, etc. Thanks Rachel, I was going round in circles until we spoke.

Writing the book became my major activity, and at times I was consumed by the effort. My partner Eileen has been just incredible during this whole time. Not only was she supporting me emotionally, she was taking up watercolor painting for the first time. Her beautiful paintings inspired me to also do something worthwhile.

Eileen has an acquaintance Cornelia Feye, another Renaissance woman, who is an editor, author and has a publishing company, Konstellation Press. Following Rachel's advice, I plowed forward, asked Cornelia if she would like to publish my book. To my happy surprise, she agreed.

She has taken the book a long way forward from the early days. Cornelia taught me that writing a story differs from telling the story, and that is a skill acquired by continuing to write. Thanks to her for going above and beyond the extra mile. Martin Hill did an outstanding job as copy editor, and bought a lot of information to the table. Finally, I want to thank all my reviewers, who were kind enough to share their time and expertise. I learned from them. that I still have a lot to learn.

And so my thanks goes to all my teachers who had the right stuff, Drs. David Streeten, John Hickam, Bill Schiess, John Sipple, Norman Levinsky, Burt Polansky, Pat Genovese, Charlie Fisch, Alan Cohen, Rory Comerford, Jim Dalen and Hugh Fulmer. Pray that some of that right stuff rubbed off on me. Looking back on the finished product, my cynicism, my irreverence, and my disrespectful attitude were not as sharp and loud as I wanted them to be, but I can still recognize my voice throughout the text.

For my parents Ben and Bea Goldberg, who sacrificed so that I might go to medical school, thanks and acknowledgement are words that fail to capture the debt and the gratitude. Honor and respect and love are the best words that I know.

Final acknowledgement to my great friend Dr. Gene Abramson. The very best physician I ever knew, and hands down, the smartest doc. His fund of knowledge was extraordinary, and hopefully some of it rubbed off on me. Alav ha shalom, Gino, I miss you.

ABOUT THE AUTHOR

Edward Lewis Goldberg began life at an early age.

His interest in the American presidents began at Cornell University, where he graduated with a major in American studies. His dream was to be a history teacher. However, following his father's strong advice, he soon found himself in medical school (Upstate Medical, Syracuse), graduated and became a physician; practiced internal medicine for over thirty years; and finally retired in 2000. Since then, he has been able to return to his love of American history, spending much of his time at the Osher programs at Brandeis, and UCSD.

Since 2020, Ed and his partner Eileen have been full time residents of San Diego, arriving just in time for Covid 19.

www.ingramcontent.com/pod-product-compliance
Lightning Source LLC
Chambersburg PA
CBHW020734020526
44118CB00033B/567